Color Science and Shade Selection in Operative Dentistry

Dayane Oliveira
Editor

Color Science and Shade Selection in Operative Dentistry

Essential Elements for Clinical Success

Springer

Editor
Dayane Oliveira
College of Dentistry
University of Florida
Gainesville, FL, USA

ISBN 978-3-030-99172-2 ISBN 978-3-030-99173-9 (eBook)
https://doi.org/10.1007/978-3-030-99173-9

This Springer imprint is published by the registered company Springer Nature Switzerland AG
The registered company address is: Gewerbestrasse 11, 6330 Cham, Switzerland

Preface

This book aims to provide information and guidance on color selection and color matching in Dentistry.

Generally speaking, color science has always been an essential and trending topic in Dentistry but never fully explored. Color science in Dentistry is usually briefly explored in book chapters. This book is looking forward to fully exploring all theories and clinical guidance to fulfill clinical success.

This book is addressed to all groups from undergraduate to postgraduate students, clinicians, and researchers. The content embraces to attend all groups but written in a way all groups can understand. The topics include the basic color science concepts till bleaching, color selection, color matching using schematic drawings, and the many different restorative techniques using resin composites and stratifications, and much more.

I appreciate all authors for their contribution to this book, their effort, and their dedication that made it all possible. It was a pleasure to collaborate with such an amazing group. Thank you so much for making this book come true!

Gainesville, FL, USA Dayane Oliveira

Contents

1 Color Science

Dayane Oliveira and Mateus Garcia Rocha

1.1 Color Definition

"Color is defined as the property of producing a visual perception as a result of the way an object reflects or emits light." Although it seems simple, color is best described as an abstract science in which it appears to be highly subjective.

In 2005, neuroscientists from University of Rochester had found that the number of color-sensitive cells in the human retina differs among people by up to 40 times; yet people appear to perceive colors the same way. These findings indicated that visual perception of color is controlled much more by the human brain than the eyes [1].

A practical example of the influence of the human brain on visual perception is shown in Fig. 1.1. Observing the square, how many shades do you see? If you see two different shades of gray, cover the line blocking the darker and lighter shading across the middle, and your brain will begin to realize that the cube actually has only one shade. This is a color illusion from Tom Cornsweet, who is best known for his work in visual perception. Color illusions are images where the surrounding colors trick the human brain into an incorrect interpretation of color [2].

Indeed, the visual perception of different colors is a subjective process whereby the brain responds to the stimuli that are produced by color-sensitive cones localized in the human retina. However, it proves the importance of color education in Dentistry [3].

1.2 Color and Its Dimensions

Color can be specified based on three color appearance parameters, also known as the three color dimensions: hue, value (or lightness), and Chroma (Fig. 1.2).

1.2.1 Hue

Hue is defined as the visual perception of the stimuli of a wavelength. As illustrated in Fig. 1.3, the main pure hues are red, blue, and yellow. The main pure hues are also called primary colors. However, the mixture of pure hues can generate different visual perception stimuli, also called secondary colors. For example, the mixture of blue (primary color) and yellow (primary color) generates the visual perception of green (secondary color). The mixture of a primary color and a secondary color can also generate a different visual perception stimulus, called a tertiary color.

D. Oliveira · M. G. Rocha (✉)
Department of Restorative Dental Sciences, College of Dentistry, University of Florida, Gainesville, FL, USA
e-mail: DOliveira@dental.ufl.edu; MRocha@dental.ufl.edu

D. Oliveira (ed.), *Color Science and Shade Selection in Operative Dentistry*,
https://doi.org/10.1007/978-3-030-99173-9_1

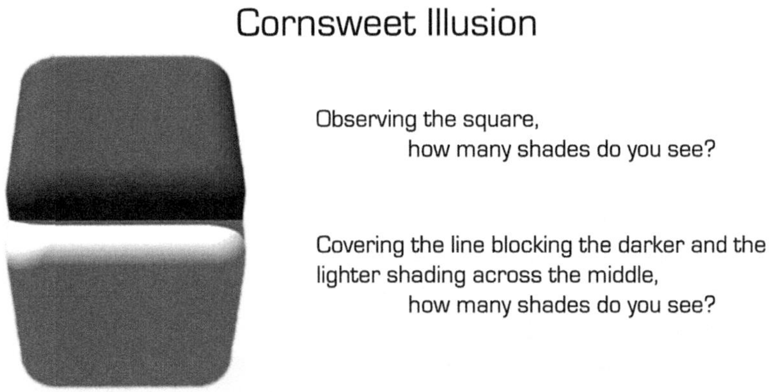

Fig. 1.1 Cornsweet illusion: color illusion designed by Tom Cornsweet

1.2.2 Value

Value, also known as lightness or tone, is referred to the lightness or darkness of a color. In other words, it indicates the quantity of the light that is reflected.

1.2.3 Chroma

Chroma is defined as the purity, intensity, or saturation of a color. Thus, a lower Chroma would indicate less intensity of the color, as in pastel colors. In contrast, a higher Chroma is related to more vivid color.

1.2.4 Translucency

Translucency is the physical property that allows light to pass through the material. The material can be considered transparent, translucent, or opaque according to the degree of light that is transmitted rather than absorbed or reflected (Fig. 1.4). When the material allows most light to pass through it, it is considered transparent. This means that it is possible to clearly see through it. On the other hand, when the material allows some light to pass through it, it is considered translucent. This means that it is still possible to see through it, but not as clearly. Last, when no light is able to pass through it, the material is considered opaque. This means that it is not possible to see through it.

Clearly, a mistake in translucency may compromise the natural appearance of a restoration in comparison to the natural teeth as the background changes. This is the reason why some authors describe translucency as the fourth dimension of color [4].

1.3 Color Perception

Color is not a property of light, but the visual perception of light by an observer. In order for the color to be perceived, three elements must be simultaneously present: illumination, an object, and an observer.

1.3.1 Light

1.3.1.1 Concepts of Illumination

Although white light is colorless to the human eye, it contains all colors in the visible wavelength spectrum (Fig. 1.5). Thus, when the white light hits an object, the different wavelengths can be absorbed, transmitted, or reflected. The reflected wavelengths will be responsible for the color perception of the object (Fig. 1.6).

However, different light sources can emit different wavelengths. This means that not all visible wavelength spectra are being absorbed, transmitted, or reflected by the object under different light sources. Thus, the color of one object can look different under different illumination.

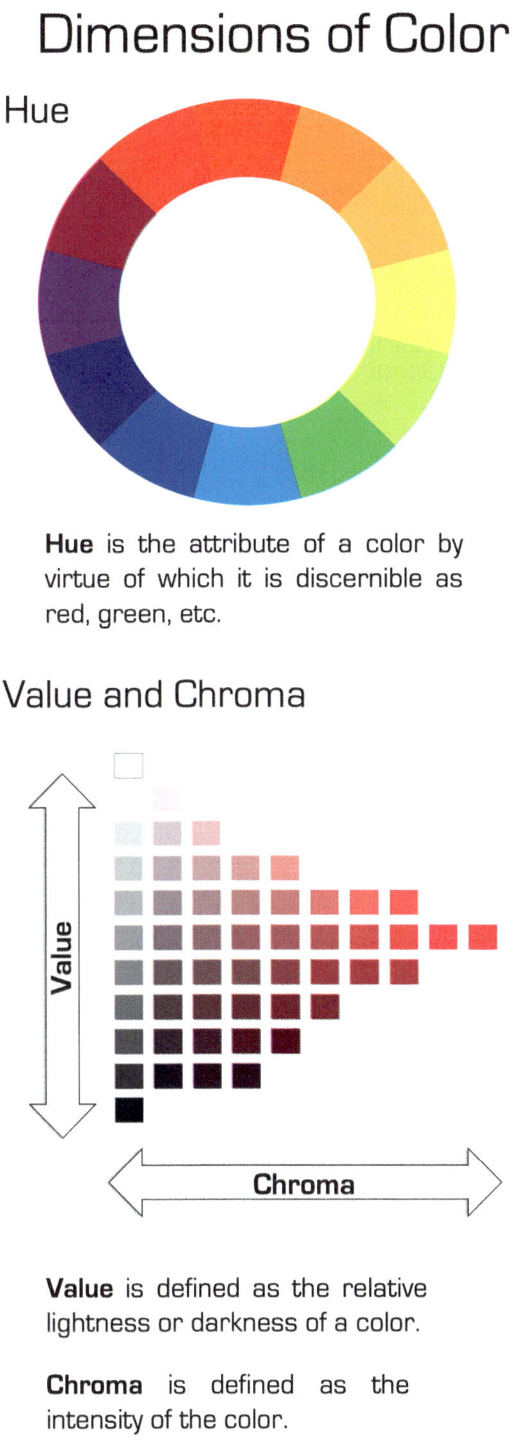

Fig. 1.2 Color dimensions: hue, value, and Chroma

1.3.2 Object

As previously explained, when the light hits an object, the different wavelengths can be absorbed, transmitted, or reflected, and the reflected wavelengths will be responsible for the color of the object (as illustrated in Fig. 1.6). It means that when the object is yellow, it absorbs and/or transmits all wavelengths, but yellow, which is reflected.

1.3.2.1 Light Reflection, Light Absorption, and Light Transmittance

> As stated by Lavoisier, in nature, nothing is created, nothing is lost, everything is transformed.

The understanding of light reflection, light absorption, and light transmittance through an object follows this rationality.

The light reflection is the change in the direction of the electromagnetic radiation at an interface between two different media. Technically, different media have different refractive indexes. The refractive index is the ratio of the speed of light in the vacuum to its speed in a specific medium. Higher the difference between the refractive indexes of the two mediums, the higher the light reflection.

Then, the amount of electromagnetic radiation that is either not reflected is absorbed or transmitted through the object. The light absorption is defined as the electromagnetic radiation energy that is transformed into the internal energy of the object (also called absorber). The reason the electromagnetic radiation is absorbed by the object while trying to pass through the object is that when it vibrates, the electrons interact with neighboring atoms in such a manner as to convert its vibrational energy into thermal energy. Thus, the light wave with that given frequency is absorbed by the object, never again released in the form of light. In contrast, the light transmittance is the electromagnetic radiation energy that was not reflected nor absorbed, being able to pass

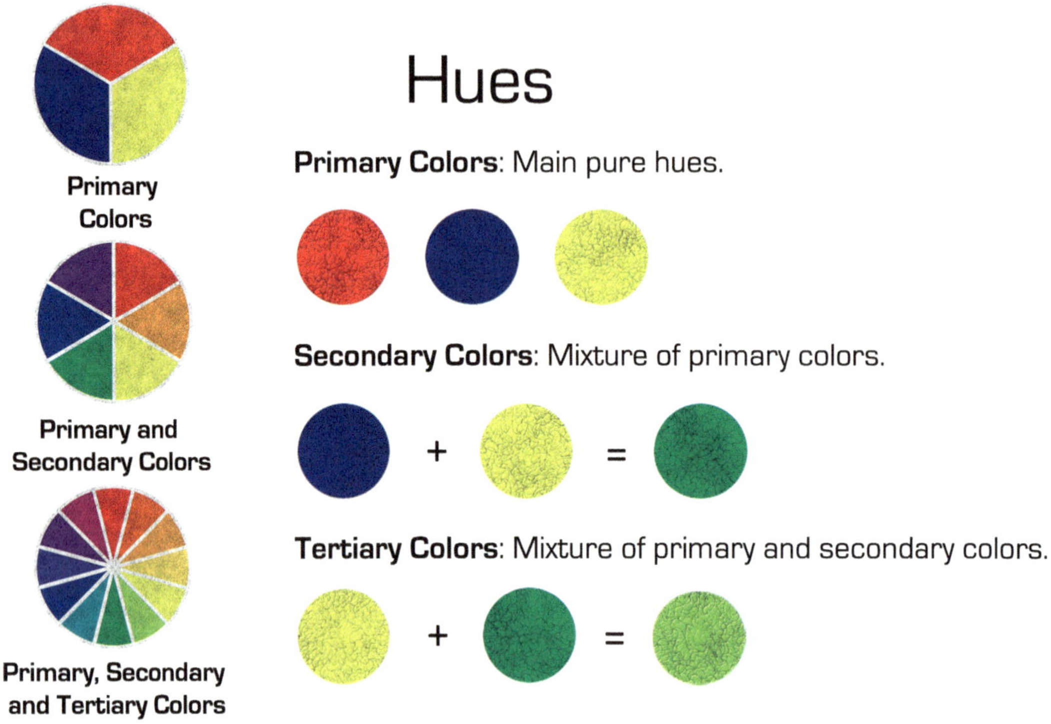

Fig. 1.3 Hues: primary, secondary, and tertiary colors

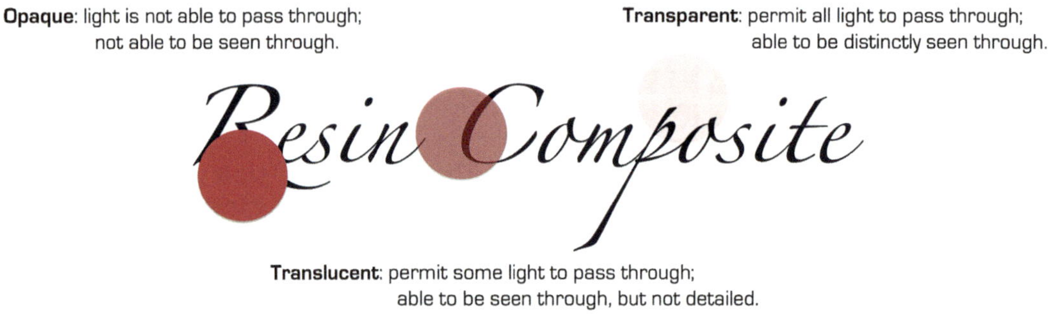

Fig. 1.4 Definition of transparency, translucency, and opacity

through the object. And in the end, how an observer perceives an object's color depends on which wavelengths are reflected by this object.

1.3.2.2 Opalescence and Counter-Opalescence

As previously mentioned, objects can be transparent, translucent, or opaque according to the degree of light that is transmitted rather than absorbed or reflected (as illustrated in Fig. 1.4). In highly translucent materials, the light that is scattered through the material can create dichroism, in which the material appears blue from the front side (opalescence), but yellowish-red shines through the backside (counter-opalescence) (Fig. 1.7). This phenomenon occurs due to a specific type of light scattering known as the Tyndall effect. Under the Tyndall effect, the longer-wavelength light, yellow-red, is more transmitted while the shorter-wavelength light, blue, is more reflected.

Enamel is a highly translucent tissue responsible for the opalescence of the incisal halo. This

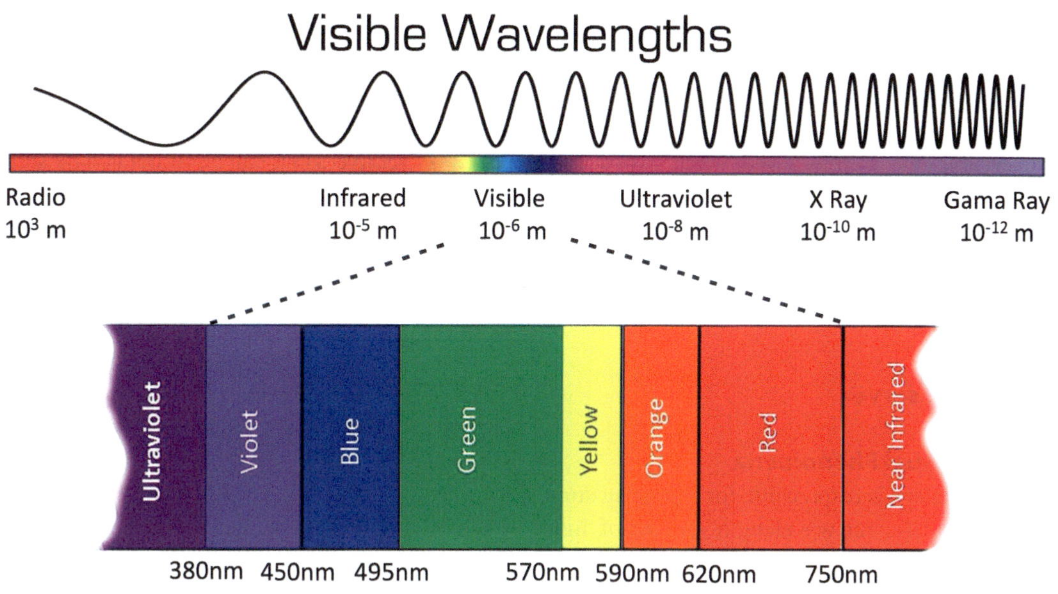

Fig. 1.5 Visible wavelength spectrums and color perception

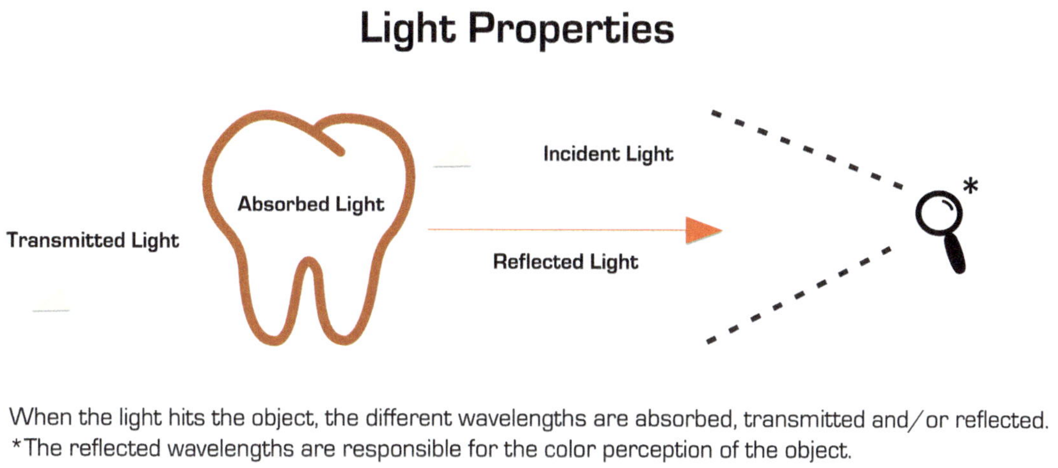

Fig. 1.6 Light absorption, reflection and transmission, and color perception

effect is not perceptible in the cervical and medium thirds of the teeth due to the presence of dentin in between, which is highly opaque [5, 6]. However, in the incisal third, it is possible to observe an opalescent halo that follows the incisal outline of the mamelon of dentin. Specific composites called "translucent" or "opalescent" can be used to reproduce this effect.

Also, the translucent multilayering characteristic of the teeth can make its color be perceived differently at different angles. This phenomenon is called goniochromism [7].

1.3.2.3 Fluorescence

On the other side, the dentin is responsible for another natural effect in the tooth: fluorescence. The fluorescence is the emission of a visible wavelength after absorption of radiation in the ultraviolet region of the spectrum, which is invisible to the human eye. Then, when exposed to ultraviolet light, the fluorescence of dentin gives a distinct color that glows. Thus, if the restorative material did not have this property, the difference between the natural teeth and the restorative material would be perceived when exposed to ultraviolet light (Fig. 1.8). However, nowadays, all dental composites have fluorescence properties due to the addition of rare earths to the composition.

1.3.3 Observer

1.3.3.1 Visual Phenomena

The human eye is responsible for capturing stimulus from different wavelength spectra of light and discharging nerve impulses that are conducted to the brain. There are three types of cone cells in the human eye that are more sensitive to either short (blue), medium (green), or long wavelengths (red) (Fig. 1.9).

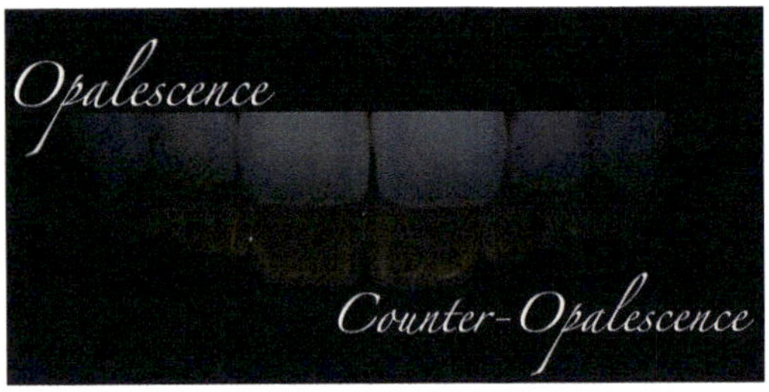

Fig. 1.7 Tyndall effect: opalescence and counter-opalescence

Despite called "blue," "green," and "red" cone cells, each type of cell does not sense only one color but a broad range of wavelengths in varying degrees of sensitivity. Because of this, different specific selective cones can be stimulated by similar wavelength spectra but in different levels. Thus, when the cone cells are exposed to a certain wavelength spectrum, the most sensitive cone cell for this specific wavelength spectrum is stimulated first.

1.3.3.2 Visual Fatigue

However, as previously mentioned, when a specific selective cone is stimulated for prolonged viewing, it causes the fatigue of these cone cells. Then, the other color receptor, which is not fatigued, receives the stimulus, and the brain incorrectly perceives the other color.

1.3.3.3 Gender

Human beings are capable of perceiving hundreds of shades equally; however, although findings are ambiguous, gender may have an influence on color perception. Thus, men and women may experience the appearance of color differently. Generally, women are expected to experience more shades of color than men. What may be simple "purple" to a man, but it could be "lavender" to a woman. Neuroscience says women are better at distinguishing among distinctions in color. On the other hand, linguistic researchers say that women possess a larger vocabulary of

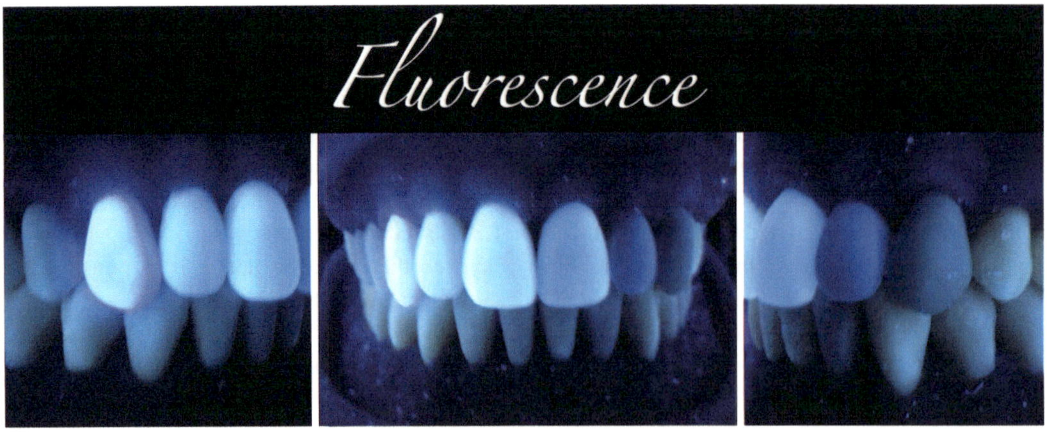

Fig. 1.8 Fluorescence effect of different composites

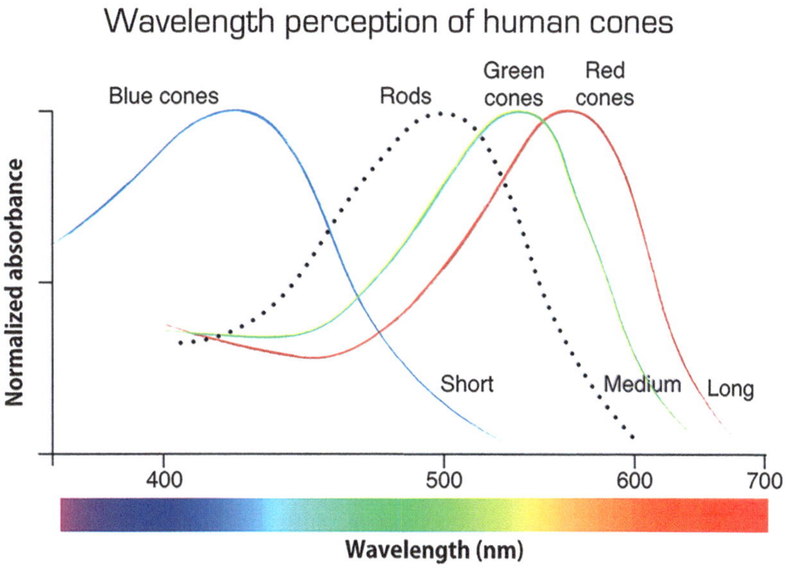

Fig. 1.9 Different wavelengths absorbance of sensory cells on human retina

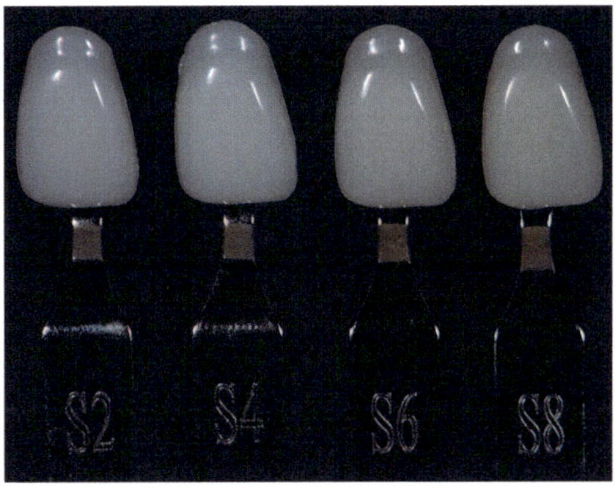

Fig. 1.10 Bleaching shade guide shades tabs with saturation in a crescent scale

shades to describe color than men. But women proved slightly better at detecting tiny differences between shades that look the same to men. The scientists believe the answer lies in the differences in men's and women's hormones that can alter development in the visual cortex. In contrast, children are more likely to sort the colors more randomly. However, the reason is probably due to the smaller exposure to color groups and general education of color [8, 9].

1.3.3.4 Expertise

As mentioned in the previous topic, exposure to color groups and general education of color directly affect how color is perceived and called. Thus, although human beings can perceive hundreds of shades equally, as more educated they are on the topic, they tend to be more attentive, percept smaller differences in nuances, and even accept those differences less. Figure 1.10 illustrates side by side different shades from a bleaching shade guide with saturation in a crescent scale; try to identify the differences in Chroma.

1.3.3.5 Age

The sensitivity of retinal cells declines with age, causing different shades of color to be less noticeable [10]. At the same time, certain neural pathways of the brain compensate it, so color perception remains constant over some time [11]. Because of this, color vision abnormalities are very uncommon in people younger than 70. However, as there is no treatment for this age-related loss of color perception, in mid-70s, dentists should be aware of this limitation.

1.3.3.6 Phenomena That Affect Color Perception

– Metamerism

  As previously explained, when the light hits an object, the different wavelengths in it can be absorbed, transmitted, or reflected. The reflected wavelengths will be responsible for the color perception of the object (as illustrated in Fig. 1.6). However, different light sources can emit different wavelengths, and the color of the object can look different under different illumination.

In some cases, the color of two different colored objects can match under one set of illumination but fail to match under a different set (Fig. 1.11). This phenomenon is known as the metamerism effect [12–14]. It shows the importance of illumination during color selection in Dentistry [15].

- Bezold–Brucke effect
  Hue perception can change as light intensity varies. This phenomenon is known as the Bezold–Brucke shift [16, 17]. As the light intensity increases, the color perception shifts more toward blue or yellow, depending on the original color of the object. Then, if the object is yellow, it tends to look more saturated than it really is (Fig. 1.12). It can influence the color selection to a more saturated color rather than the original color of the teeth. At lower intensities, however, the color perception shifts more toward the red/green axis.
- Stiles–Crawford Effect
  The Stiles–Crawford effect is the phenomenon where light reaching the eye near the edge of the pupil produces a lower photoreceptor response compared to light of similar intensity reaching the eye near the center of the pupil. This phenomenon is so vital in Dentistry because teeth color is multichromatic, and depending on the angle that the color is observed, color perception can vary [18].
- Aubert or Abney Effect
  The Aubert or Abney effect is also known as the purity-on-hue effect. This effect described the perceived hue shift that occurs when white light is added to a monochromatic light source. The addition of white light causes a desaturation of the monochromatic light, as perceived by the human eye. For this reason, this hue

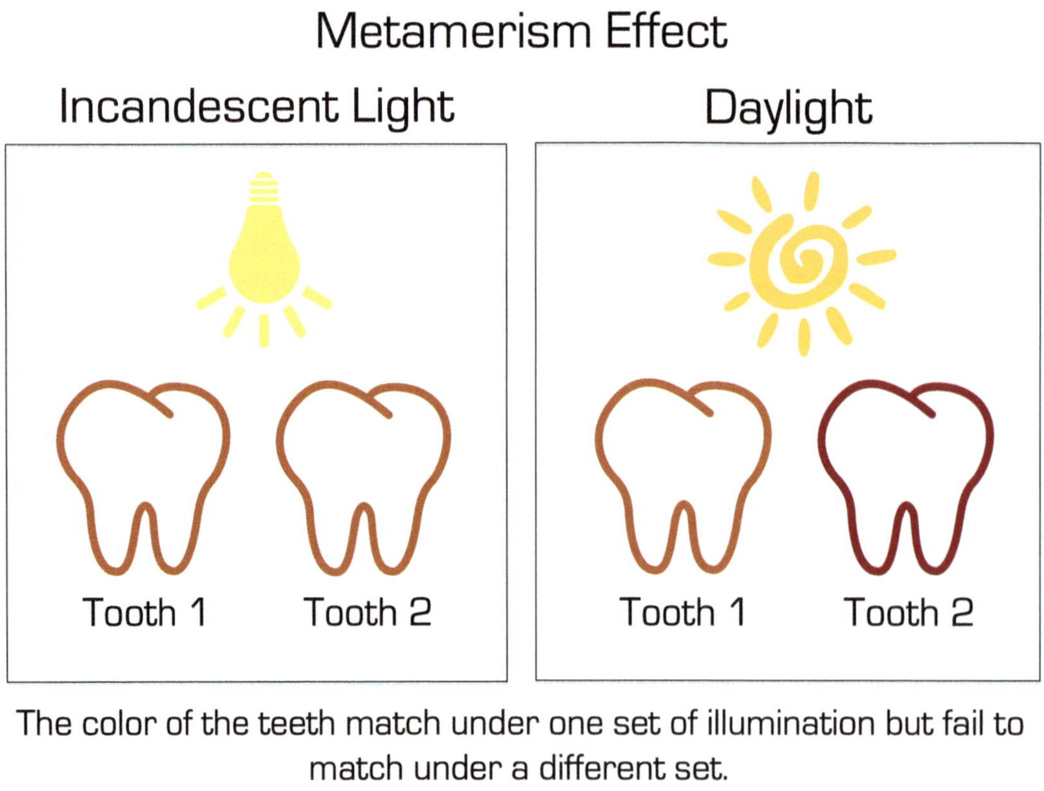

Fig. 1.11 Metamerism phenomenon

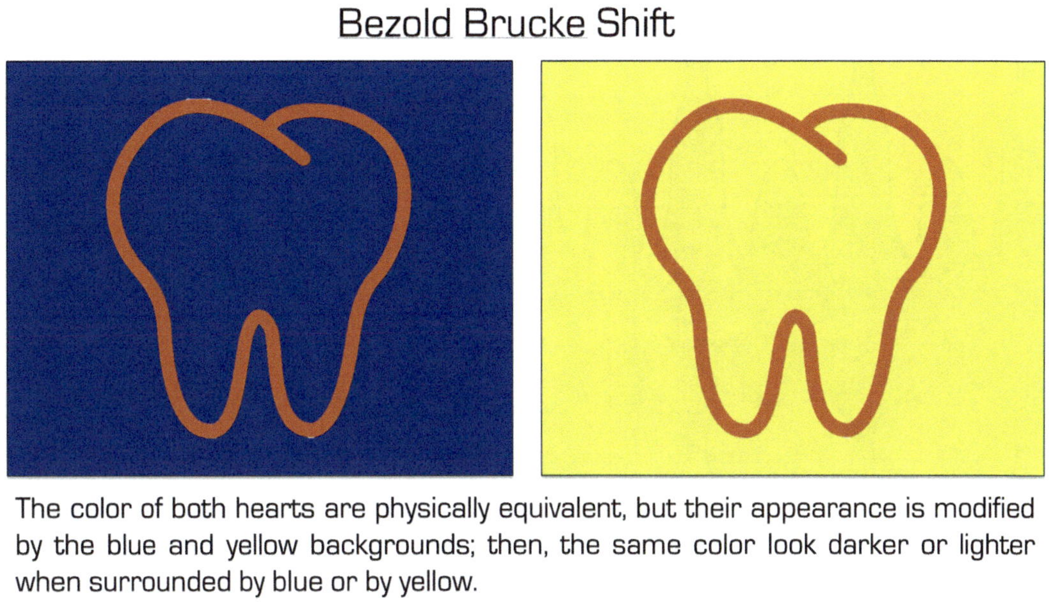

Fig. 1.12 Bezold–Brucke phenomenon

shift phenomenon is considered more a physiological effect than a physical effect [19].

– Helmholtz–Kohlrausch Effect
  The Helmholtz–Kohlrausch effect is another physiological effect in which colored light appears brighter than white light of the same luminance [20]. This phenomenon can also be observed in colored pigments and printing, although less pronounced. When the colors are more saturated, the human eye interprets it as the color's luminance and Chroma, thus tricking the brain into believing that the colors are brighter (Fig. 1.13).

  Notice that brightness and lightness are different concepts. Brightness is the intensity of the object regardless of the light source. Lightness is the brightness of the object with respect to the light reflecting on it. An exception to this is when the human observed is red–green colorblind, thus not being able to distinguish differences between the lightness of the colors.

– Opponent-Color Theory
  The human eyes receive stimulus from different wavelengths by different sensory cells on the retina, the cones. There are specific selective cones for different wavelength ranges. However, when a specific selective cone is stimulated for prolonged viewing, it causes the fatigue of these cone cells. Then, the opponent-color receptor, which is not fatigued, receives the stimulus, and the brain incorrectly perceives the opponent color. This phenomenon is known as the opponent-color theory.

  This phenomenon can be observed in Dentistry. As the rubber dam is usually brightly colored, it may alter the color perception of the tooth and lead to an incorrect color selection. This is the reason why shade selection should be made before the dam is applied [4]. Otherwise, prolonged exposure to the bright color of the dam can desensitize a specific selective cone and stimulate the opponent's specific selective cone when trying to select the color of the tooth

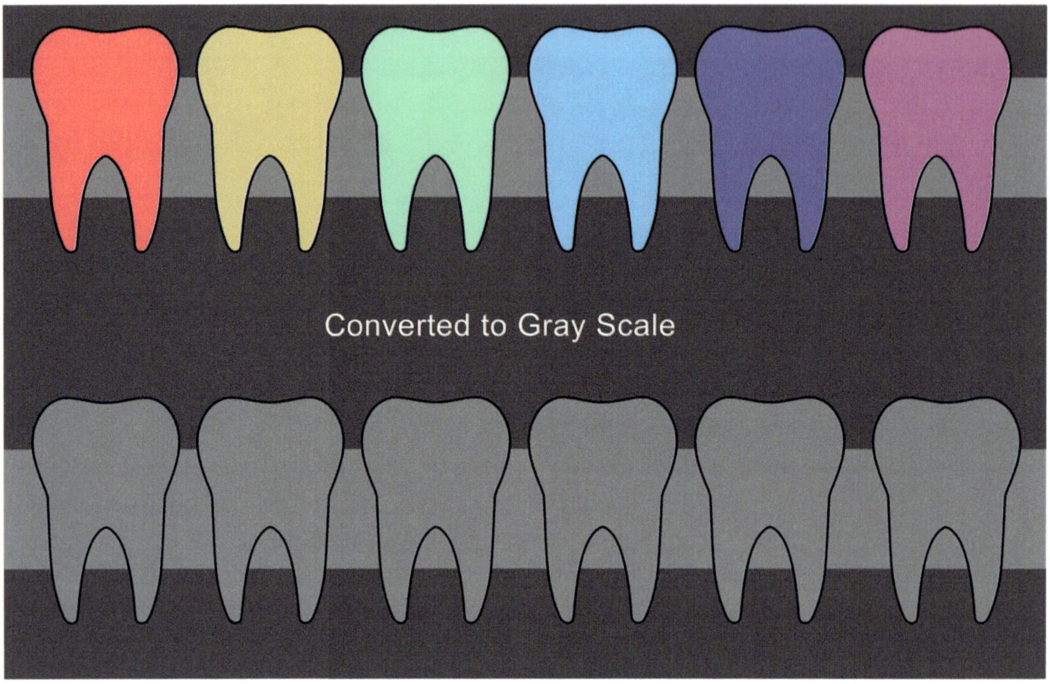

Fig. 1.13 Helmholtz–Kohlrausch effect

under absolute operatory field isolation. The opponent colors are blue and yellow, red and green, and black and white (Fig. 1.14). Toward a better understanding of this theory, a practical example is given in Fig. 1.15.

It is worthwhile to mention that the absolute operatory field isolation also causes the dehydration of the teeth. Natural teeth exhibit high gloss reflection when wet. Thus, the color appearance looks vivid. However, in the absence of saliva, the roughness of the teeth surface scatters the light, and the color appearance looks more pastel.

– Von Kries Law

Chromatic adaptation the human visual ability to adjust to changes in illumination in order to preserve the appearance of object colors. Various theories explain the color constancy phenomena under illuminant changes. The Von Kries law describes the relationship between the illuminant and human visual system sensitivity [21].

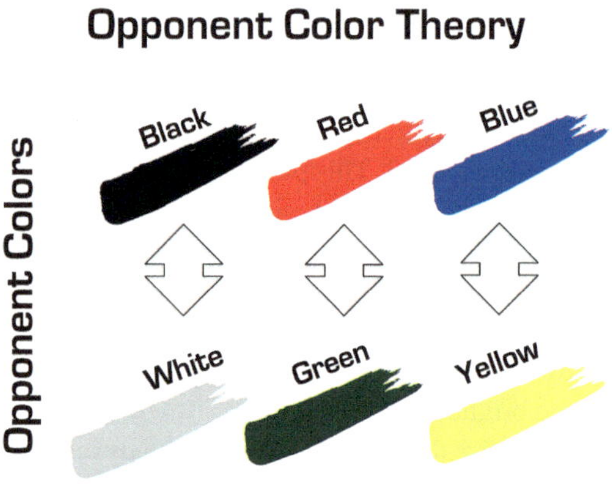

Fig. 1.14 Opponent-color theory: opponent colors

The Von Kries law is frequently used in-camera image processing. Cameras with no adjustments for light may register color differently. Thus, a correction, also known as white balance, is used to simulate this feature of chromatic adaptation by the human eye.

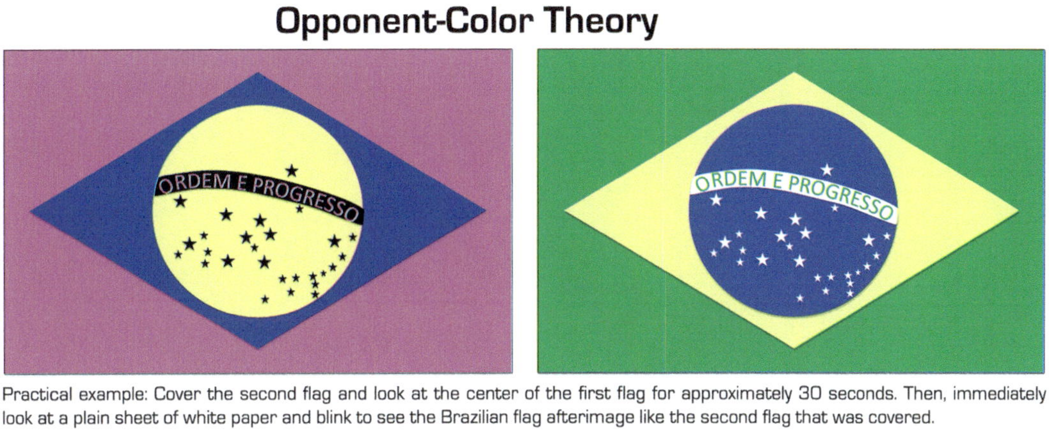
Opponent-Color Theory
ORDEM E PROGRESSO
ORDEM E PROGRESSO
Practical example: Cover the second flag and look at the center of the first flag for approximately 30 seconds. Then, immediately look at a plain sheet of white paper and blink to see the Brazilian flag afterimage like the second flag that was covered.

Fig. 1.15 Opponent-color theory test: practical example

References

1. Hofer H, Carroll J, Neitz J, Neitz M, Williams DR. Organization of the human trichromatic cone mosaic. J Neurosci. 2005;25(42):9669–79.
2. Cornsweet T. Visual perception. New York: Academic Press; 1970.
3. Ristic I, Stankovic S, Paravina RD. Influence of color education and training on shade matching skills. J Esthet Restor Dent. 2016;28(5):287–94.
4. Dudea D, Gasparik C, Botos A, Alb F, Irimie A, Paravina RD. Influence of background/surrounding area on accuracy of visual color matching. Clin Oral Investig. 2016;20(6):1167–73.
5. Pop-Ciutrila IS, Ghinea R, Perez Gomez Mdel M, Colosi HA, Dudea D, Badea M. Dentin scattering, absorption, transmittance and light reflectivity in human incisors, canines and molars. J Dent. 2015;43(9):1116–24.
6. Pop-Ciutrila IS, Ghinea R, Colosi HA, Dudea D. Dentin translucency and color evaluation in human incisors, canines, and molars. J Prosthet Dent. 2016;115(4):475–81.
7. Chirdon WM, O'Brien WJ, Robertson RE. Mechanisms of gonochromism relevant to restorative dentistry. Dent Mater. 2009;25(6):802–9.
8. Abramov I, Gordon J, Feldman O, Chavarga A. Sex & vision I: spatio-temporal resolution. Biol Sex Differ. 2012;3(1):20.
9. Abramov I, Gordon J, Feldman O, Chavarga A. Sex & vision II: color appearance of monochromatic lights. Biol Sex Differ. 2012;3(1):21.
10. Haegerstrom-Portnoy G, Schneck ME, Lott LA, Hewlett SE, Brabyn JA. Longitudinal increase in anisometropia in older adults. Optom Vis Sci. 2014;91(1):60–7.
11. Wueger S. Colour constancy across the life span: evidence for compensatory mechanisms. PLoS One. 2013;8(5):e63921.
12. Feng X, Xu W, Han Q, Zhang S. LED light with enhanced color saturation and improved white light perception. Opt Express. 2016;24(1):573–85.
13. Kim SH, Lee YK, Lim BS, Rhee SH, Yang HC. Metameric effect between dental porcelain and porcelain repairing resin composite. Dent Mater. 2007;23(3):374–9.
14. Akbarinia A, Gegenfurtner KR. Color metamerism and the structure of illuminant space. J Opt Soc Am A Opt Image Sci Vis. 2018;35(4):231–8.
15. Clary JA, Ontiveros JC, Cron SG, Paravina RD. Influence of light source, polarization, education and training on shade matching quality. J Prosthet Dent. 2016;116(1):91–7.
16. Imhoff SM, Volbrecht VJ, Nerger JL. A new look at the Bezold–Brucke hue shift in the peripheral retina. Vis Res. 2004;44(16):1891–906.
17. Pridmore RW. Bezold–Brucke hue-shift as functions of luminance level, luminance ratio, interstimulus interval and adapting white for aperture and object colors. Vis Res. 1999;39(23):3873–91.
18. Westheimer G. Retinal light distributions, the stiles-Crawford effect and apodization. J Opt Soc Am A Opt Image Sci Vis. 2013;30(7):1417–21.
19. Kurtenbach W, Sternheim CE, Spillmann L. Change in hue of spectral colors by dilution with white light (Abney effect). J Opt Soc Am A. 1984;1(4):365–72.
20. Corney D, Haynes JD, Rees G, Lotto RB. The brightness of colour. PLoS One. 2009;4(3):e5091.
21. MacAdam DL. Chromatic adaptation. In: Color measurement. Springer series in optical sciences, vol. 27. Berlin: Springer; 1985.

Natural Tooth X Composites Biomimetics

2

Dayane Oliveira, Rodrigo Rocha Maia,
and André Figueiredo Reis

2.1 Optical Properties of the Natural Tooth

The tooth color is determined by the absorption and reflection of the incident light in the different natural tooth structures: the enamel and the dentin [1, 2]. These tissues have different structural characteristics and, consequently, exhibit different optical properties (Fig. 2.1).

2.1.1 Composition of the Natural Tooth Structures

2.1.1.1 Enamel

The enamel is composed of inorganic and organic components. The inorganic part is hydroxyapatite, 96% mineral by weight, and more than 86% by volume is hydroxyapatite. The hydroxyapatite crystals are colorless and organized in a hierarchical and organized way above the dentin. The organic constituents are 4–12% by volume water, included in the intercrystalline spaces and a network of micropores opening to the external surface. These microchannels allow a dynamic connection between the oral cavity outside and the dentin underneath the enamel. These characteristics give the enamel a slight whitish color look with high translucency [2].

2.1.1.2 Dentin

Dentin is a unique mineralized avascular connective tissue. It constitutes a hydrated biological tissue—composed of 70% inorganic material, 18% organic material, and 12% water, by weight—whose structural properties and components vary according to the area analyzed. Its inorganic part consists of crystals of hydroxyapatite, while the organic portion contains mainly type I collagen and fractions of type III and V collagen, glycoproteins and proteoglycans, non-collagen proteins, and water [1]. Different from the enamel, the dentin is not colorless; its hue naturally varies among yellow, orange, and brown shades with low translucency. Also, the low translucency of the dentin compared to the high translucency of the enamel is due to the lower amount of inorganic content and increased amount of organic content.

2.1.1.3 Dentin–Enamel Junction (DEJ)

The dentin–enamel junction (DEJ) is a thin layer constituted of partially mineralized collagen protein fiber bundles in between the enamel and the

D. Oliveira · A. F. Reis
Department of Restorative Dental Sciences, College of Dentistry, University of Florida, Gainesville, FL, USA
e-mail: DOliveira@dental.ufl.edu; AReis@dental.ufl.edu

R. R. Maia (✉)
Department of Cariology, Restorative Sciences and Endodontics, School of Dentistry, University of Michigan, Ann Arbor, MI, USA
e-mail: rmaia@umich.edu

D. Oliveira (ed.), *Color Science and Shade Selection in Operative Dentistry*,
https://doi.org/10.1007/978-3-030-99173-9_2

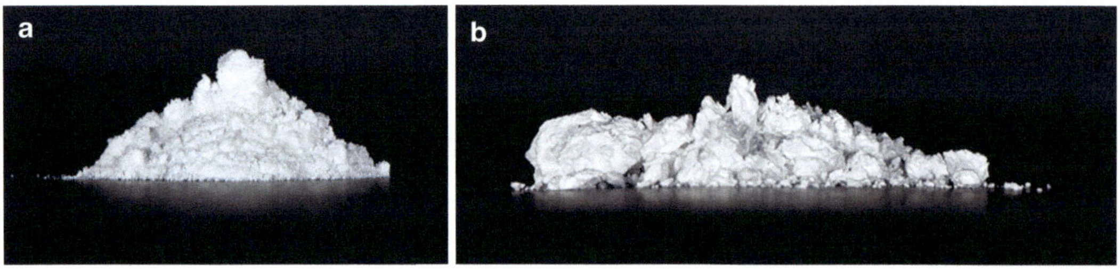

Fig. 2.3 Dental filler particles used in the composition of resin composites: (**a**) silica and (**b**) glass

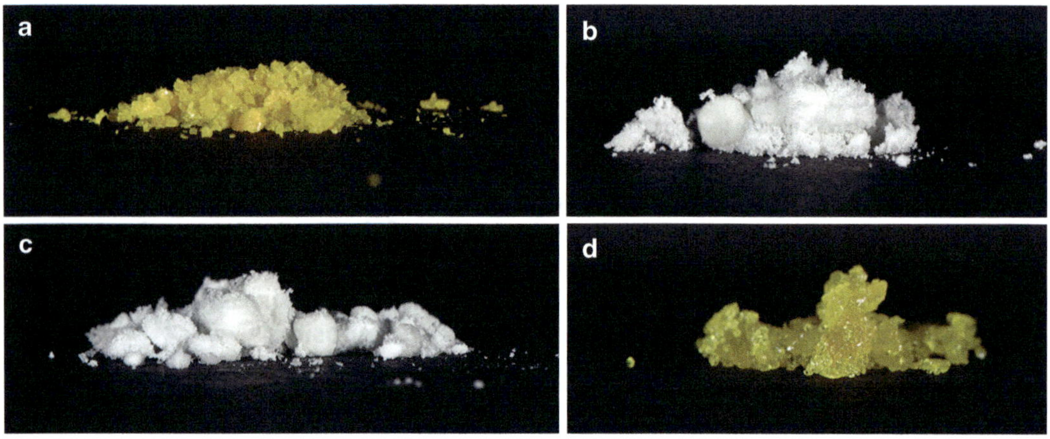

Fig. 2.4 Dental photoinitiators: (**a**) camphorquinone; (**b**) BAPO; (**c**) TPO; (**d**) ivocerin

2.2.1.2 Fillers

The inorganic portion of the resin composites, on the other hand, consists of particles of quartz (SiO_2), silica (SiO_2), zirconia (ZrO_2), barium aluminosilicate ($BaO{\cdot}Al_2O_3{\cdot}2SiO_2$), or a combination of these particles [6]. All these filler particles are whitish powders (Fig. 2.4). The different particles or their combination can be used according to the type of monomers used in the formulation of the resin composite. The reason for this is because all different monomers and filler particles have different refractive indexes.

As previously explained in Chap. 1, the refractive index is the ratio of the speed of light in the vacuum to its speed in a specific medium. Higher the difference between the refractive indexes of the two mediums, the higher the light reflection. Thus, the type and amount of these components can affect the way the light is reflected, absorbed, or transmitted [7], thus affecting its color perception. It is important to mention that the manufacturers can also use different filler particle sizes to adjust this variable. However, it is known that better polishing, lower surface roughness, and higher gloss retention are achieved with smaller particles [8–10]. The reason is that when white light shines on any solid, some of the light is directly reflected from the surface and remains white. However, most of it is absorbed and transmitted, reflecting only a few wavelengths giving the perception of the color of the object. As a result, an extremely rough surface appears lighter than a smooth surface of the same material. The reason is that most of the white light will be directly reflected from the surface. This problem is associated with unpolished composite restorations that appear lighter and less chromatic (grayer) before polishing [5].

2.2.1.3 Coupling Agent

Coupling agents are meant to link dissimilar materials. As previously described, the resin composites are composed of an organic portion, the monomers, and an inorganic portion, the fillers. However, organic and inorganic molecules do not have any interaction or adhesion in between each other. For this reason, an organosilane is used as a coupling agent in the composition of resin composites [6]. The organosilane contains an organic portion in one of its ends which bonds to the monomers. While, on the other end, the organosilane has a silane that bonds to the hydroxyl groups of the filler. Similar to the monomers, the organosilanes are colorless liquids. The organosilane liquid is pre-applied to the surface of the filler particles before mixed with the monomers.

2.2.1.4 Photoinitiators

The photoinitiator is the component added to the material that makes it light-curable. The photoinitiator is a molecule that when absorbs light, generating free radicals that initiate the polymerization process. Most composites are light-activated within the blue wavelength spectrum (420–495 nm) using a diketone as a photoinitiator, the camphorquinone (CQ). However, CQ is a yellowed-colored powder (Fig. 2.5a) that can directly interfere with the color of the resin composite, especially regarding lighter and more translucent colors. For this reason, some manufacturers use alternative photoinitiators, such as the bisalkyl phosphine oxide (BAPO) (Fig. 2.5b) and the monoalkyl phosphine oxide (TPO) (Fig. 2.5c) that are whited-colored powders [10]. It is worthwhile to mention that Ivocerin is slightly less yellow than CQ, but still, a yellowed-colored powder (Fig. 2.5d) that can also interfere with the color of the resin composite [10].

These colorful photoinitiators also interfere with the color matching between the resin composite and the tooth. After absorbing its corresponding wavelength, it reacts and is consumed. After its consumption, the material becomes less yellow. For this reason, it is recommended to light-cure small increments of different shades of the resin composite on top of the tooth to better select color. This technique will be further explored and explained in Chap. 3.

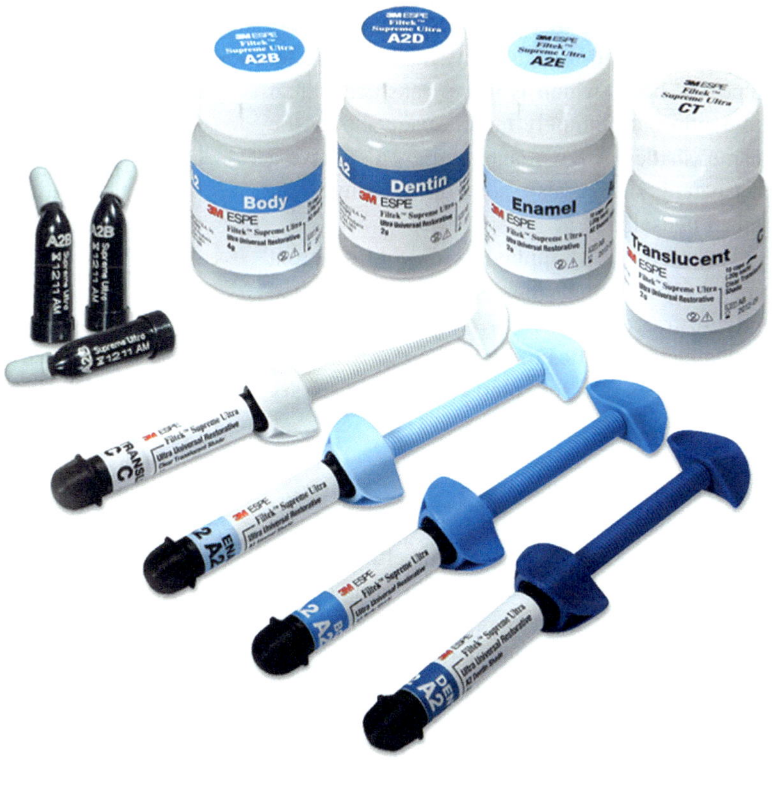

Fig. 2.5 Resin composite with different translucencies: (**a**) dentin; (**b**) body; (**c**) enamel; (**d**) incisal. (*Photography courtesy of 3M*)

2.2.1.5 Pigments

The pigment is the component added to the material to characterize its final color [6]. As previously explained, all the resin composite components have different colors that can interfere with the final color appearance of the material. For this reason, different pigments can be added accordingly to produce the different shades usually needed in Dentistry. The most common pigments used in dental resin composites are iron oxides (red or yellow) and titanium dioxides (white).

2.2.2 Optical Properties

2.2.2.1 Translucency

As previously explained, the dentin and the enamel have different translucencies. The enamel is more translucent, while the dentin is opaquer. Thus, mimicking these different optical properties requires different types of resin composites [11, 12]. Most manufacturers have at least two types of translucencies for their resin composites, conveniently named dentin (opaquer) and enamel (more translucent) shades. Other manufacturers also have a mid-translucency material shade, named as body, which is more translucent than the dentin but definitely much opaquer than the enamel shades. A few manufacturers also have a transparent shade, also sometimes convenient named incisal.

The techniques applied with the different types of resin composites are further described and illustrated in Chap. 7. Depending on the tooth's characteristics to be restored, a single or multiple types of resin composites are necessary to achieve perfect biomimetics [13–17].

2.2.2.2 Fluorescence

As previously mentioned, the dentin and the enamel have a natural fluorescent effect on the tooth. In the composition of resin composites, rare earths are added to reproduce this effect artificially. However, although, nowadays, all resin composites have fluorescence properties, their intensities can vary depending on the concentration of the rare earths added (see Fig. 1.8, Chap. 1). Even different natural teeth might have different fluorescence intensities due to differences in dentin and enamel composition and thicknesses [18, 19]. Still, some brands have a more similar fluorescence effect to most natural teeth than others [20].

2.2.2.3 Opalescence and Counter-Opalescence

In highly translucent materials, the light that is scattered through the material can create dichroism, in which the material appears blue from the front side (opalescence), but yellowish-red shines through the backside (counter-opalescence). The natural enamel is a highly translucent tissue responsible for the opalescence of the incisal halo. The composites described before as translucent or incisal can be used to reproduce this effect. For this reason, some manufacturers also call this type of resin composite opalescent.

References

1. Sulieman MAM. An overview of tooth-bleaching techniques: chemistry, safety and efficacy. Periodontology. 2000;48(1):148–96.
2. Ferraris F, Diamantopoulou S, Acunzo R, Alcidi R. Influence of enamel composite thickness on value, chroma and translucency of a high and a nonhigh refractive index resin composite. Int J Esthet Dent. 2014;9(3):382–401.
3. Brodbelt RH, O'Brien WJ, Fan PL, Frazer-Dib JG, Yu R. Translucency of human dental enamel. J Dent Res. 1981;60(10):1749–53.
4. Spitzer D, Bosch JT. The absorption and scattering of light in bovine and human dental enamel. Calcif Tissue Res. 1975;17(2):129–37.
5. Baratieri LN, Araujo E, Monteiro S Jr. Color in natural teeth and direct resin composite restorations: essential aspects. Eur J Esthet Dent. 2007;2(2):172–86.
6. Craig RG, Sakaguchi RL, Powers JM. Craig's restorative dental materials. Br Dent J. 2013;213(2):90.
7. Shortall AC, Palim WM, Burtscher P. Refractive index mismatch and monomer reactivity influence composite curing depth. J Dent Res. 2008;87(1):84–8.
8. Da Costa J, Ferracane J, Paravina RD, Mazur RF, Roeder L. The effect of different polishing systems on surface roughness and gloss of various resin composites. J Esthet Restor Dent. 2007;19:214–24. https://doi.org/10.1111/j.1708-8240.2007.00104.x.
9. O'Neill C, Kreplak L, Rueggeberg FA, Labrie D, Shimokawa CAK, Price RB. Effect of tooth brushing on gloss retention and surface roughness of five

bulk-fill resin composites. J Esthet Restor Dent. 2018;30:59–69. https://doi.org/10.1111/jerd.12350.
10. De Oliveira DC, Rocha MG, Gattia A, Correr AB, Ferracane JL, Sinhoreti MA. Effect of different photoinitiators and reducing agents on cure efficiency and color stability of resin-based composites using different LED wavelengths. J Dent. 2015;43(12):1565–72.
11. Villarroel M, Fahl N, De Sousa AM, De Oliveira OB Jr. Direct esthetic restorations based on translucency and opacity of composite resins. J Esthet Restor Dent. 2011;23(2):73–87.
12. Maia R, De Oliveira DC, D'Antonio T, Qian F, Skiff F. Double-layer build-up technique: laser evaluation of light propagation in dental substrates and dental composites. Int J Esthet Dent. 2018;13(4):1–14.
13. Fahl N Jr. Single-shaded direct anterior composite restorations: a simplified technique for enhanced results. Compend Contin Educ Dent. 2012;33(2):150–4.
14. Dietschi D. Free-hand bonding in the esthetic treatment of anterior teeth: creating the illusion. J Esthet Dent. 1997;9(4):156–64.
15. Ardu S, Krejci I. Biomimetic direct composite stratification technique for the restoration of anterior teeth. (Erratum in: Quintessence Int. 2006 May;37(5):408). Quintessence Int. 2006;37(3):167–74.
16. Dietschi D, Ardu S, Krejci I. A new shading concept based on natural tooth color applied to direct composite restorations. Quintessence Int. 2006;37(2):91–102.
17. Fahl N Jr. Achieving ultimate anterior esthetics with a new microhybrid composite. Compend Contin Educ Dent Suppl. 2000;26:4–13.
18. Pop-Ciutrila IS, Ghinea R, del Perez Gomez MM, Colosi HA, Dudea D, Badea M. Dentin scattering, absorption, transmittance and light reflectivity in human incisors, canines and molars. J Dent. 2015;43(9):1116–24.
19. Pop-Ciutrila IS, Ghinea R, Colosi HA, Dudea D. Dentin translucency and color evaluation in human incisors, canines, and molars. J Prosthet Dent. 2016;115(4):475–81.
20. Chirdon WM, O'Brien WJ, Robertson RE. Mechanisms of goniochromism relevant to restorative dentistry. Dent Mater. 2009;25(6):802–9.

3 Color Selection in Operative Dentistry

Vinícius Salgado and Dayane Oliveira

3.1 Illumination

As previously explained in Chap. 1, different light sources contain different wavelengths. This means that the color of the same object can be perceived differently under different illuminations.

People are usually exposed to light sources during their routine: daylight, shade or cloudy sky, fluorescent light, incandescent light, etc. These different light sources have different color temperatures. The color temperature is related to the color appearance of the light emitted by the light source.

3.1.1 Color Temperature

The color temperature is expressed in Kelvin (K). Color temperatures over 5000 K are called cool colors (blueish white), while lower color temperatures are called warm colors (yellowish white). Daylight, fluorescent light, incandescent light, for example, are warm colors, while the shade and cloudy sky are cooler colors (Fig. 3.1). Thus, the same object can have its color distorted when exposed to light sources with different color temperatures.

While low light intensity can affect hue perception, the high light intensity can cause glare and result in fatigue to the eyes. In Dentistry, the recommended standard for color selection is a color temperature of 5500 K, which corresponds to the ideal natural daylight. However, natural light conditions vary from 3000 to 8000 K depending on the time (sunrise/sunshine) and the weather (sunny/cloudy). A practical way to have more color matching success regardless of the natural conditions is to use a standardizing daylight lamp in the dental office. However, portable light-correcting devices are also available to assist chairside shade matching.

3.1.2 Light-Correcting Devices

Portable light-correcting devices were designed to assist chairside shade matching in Dentistry (Fig. 3.2). These devices consist of a ring with a window-hole that enables viewing the patient's teeth. The ring is attached to an ergonomic handle that allows the dentist to get very close to the patients' teeth. Inside the window-hole, LEDs simulating different illumination conditions. The different LEDs are disposed of so that the teeth are illuminated equally from all directions to avoid glare, distortion, and reflection.

V. Salgado (✉)
Private Practice, Rio de Janeiro, RJ, Brazil

D. Oliveira
Department of Restorative Dental Sciences, College of Dentistry, University of Florida, Gainesville, FL, USA
e-mail: DOliveira@dental.ufl.edu

D. Oliveira (ed.), *Color Science and Shade Selection in Operative Dentistry*,
https://doi.org/10.1007/978-3-030-99173-9_3

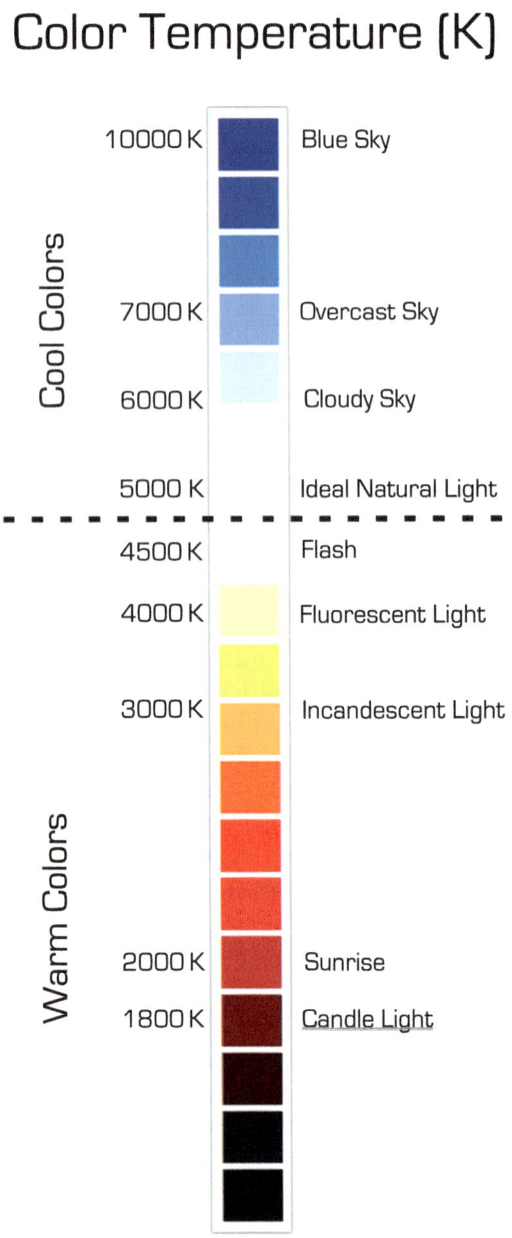

Fig. 3.1 Cool colors and warm colors: color temperature of different light sources

Both devices contain LEDs with 5500 K color temperature simulating the outdoor daylight. Other LEDs simulate indoor ambient light from halogen and incandescent light sources.

These devices also have a polarizing filter that eliminates reflection and enhance the visualization of internal details of the teeth (Fig. 3.3). It is worthwhile to mention that the use of a polarizing filter does not help shade matching. But it can help achieve shade matching by identifying internal details of the teeth for future characterization and layering [1, 2].

3.2 Color Selection Methods for Composite Restorations

Color selection is the first step before restoring a tooth. Different methods are described in the literature to select color in Dentistry. These methods are mainly categorized as subjective methods (more commonly known as visual methods) or objectives methods. The most traditionally used method is the visual analysis of color.

3.2.1 Visual Methods

The color of teeth is mainly subjectively measured by the visual comparison method using a shade guide tab, or material increments placed close or onto the tooth surface [3].

3.2.1.1 Using Shade Guides for Ceramics

The *Vitapan Classical* shade guide (VITA Zahnfabrik) is the most used shade guide in worldwide clinical practice. Introduced in 1983, it is based on VITA previous shade guide, *Lumin-VACUUM* (which was introduced in 1956). It has 16 different acrylic shade tabs empirically organized by the manufacturer (Fig. 3.4). Each tab has cervical, body, and incisal colors over an opaque background, and it is identified and named according to the body shade. The color range is divided into four different hue groups designated by *A*, *B*, *C*, and *D* letters, representing reddish–brownish for *A* hue, reddish–yellowish for *B* hue, grayish for *C* hue, and reddish–gray for *D* hue. For each hue group, there are different tabs differentiated by an Arabic number ranging from 1 to 4, with different Chromas and values. The higher the number, the higher Chroma and the lower the value. The tabs of the Vita Classical shade guide can also be repositioned in value

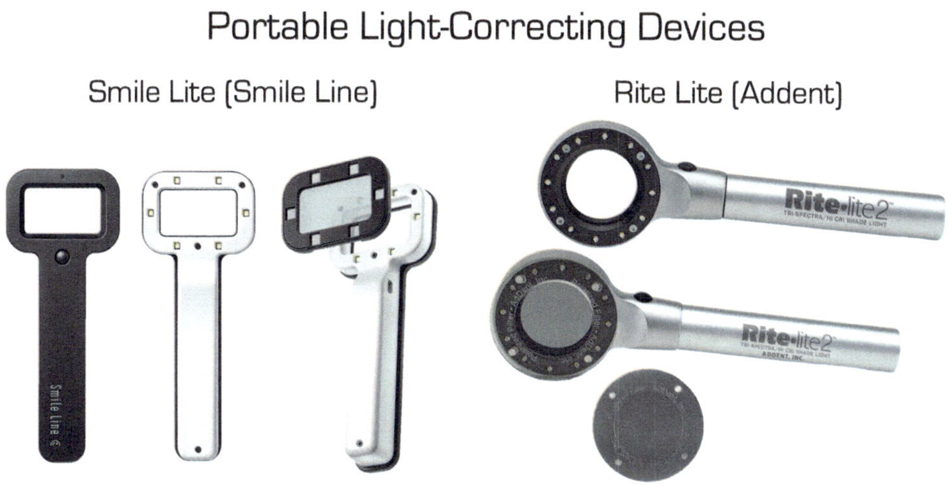

Fig. 3.2 Portable light-correcting devices: Smile Lite (Styleitaliano) and Rite Lite (Addent)

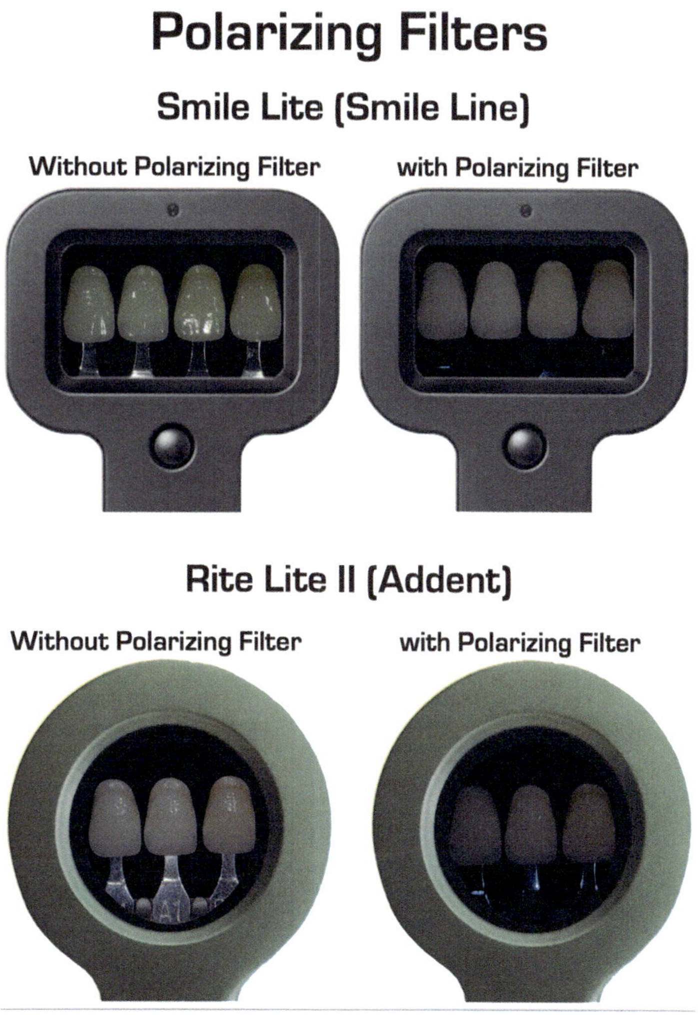

Fig. 3.3 Details' perception using light-correcting devices with and without polarizing filters

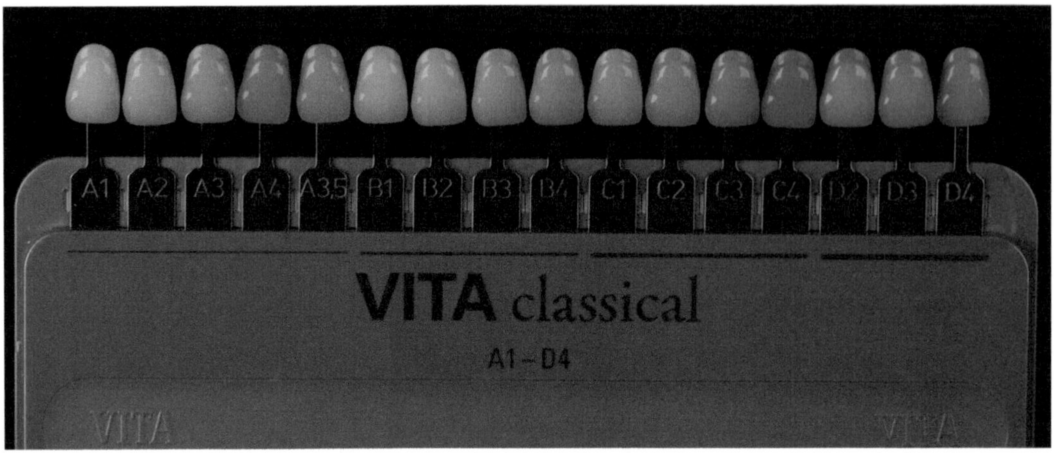

Fig. 3.4 Ceramic shade guides: *Vitapan Classical* (VITA Zahnfabrik)

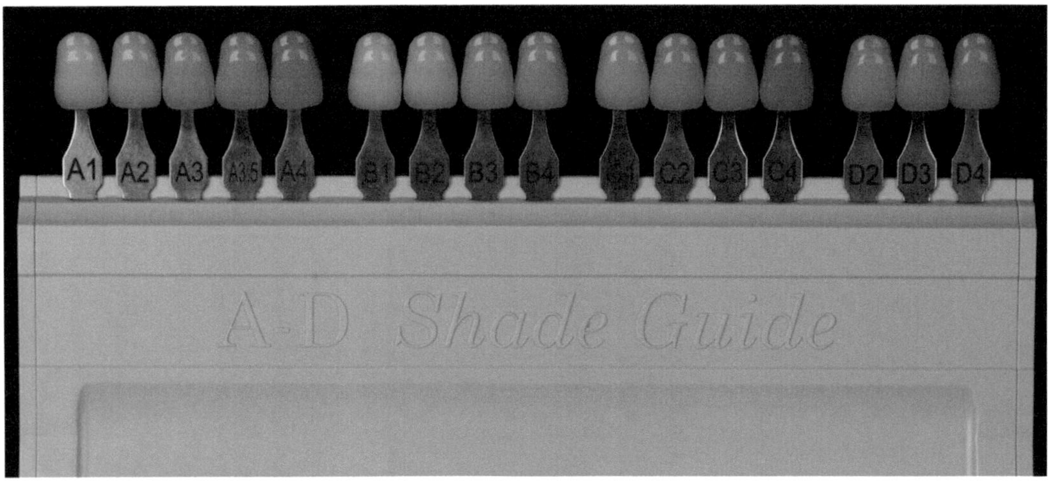

Fig. 3.5 Ceramic shade guides: *Noritake* (Kuraray Noritake)

order: B1, A1, B2, D2, A2, C1, C2, D4, A3, D3, B3, A3.5, B4, C3, A4, C4. In this way, the tabs will be reordered from the brighter to the darker shade.

There are other shade guides designed for ceramic restorations that follow the *Vitapan Classical* color distribution concept. The *A–D* shade guide (Ivoclar Vivadent) is the common color standard for Ivoclar Vivadent ceramics (Fig. 3.5). It also has 16 different acrylic shade tabs. The *Noritake* shade guide (Kuraray Noritake) is the color standard for Noritake ceramics (Fig. 3.6). It contains 20 different shade tabs, 16 based on *Vitapan Classical* color concept and 4 original shade tabs (NW0, NW0.5, NP1.5, and NP2.5). The NP hue corresponds to the slightly reddish shades than VITA *A* hue. The NP1.5 Chroma is between A1 and A2 shades while the NP2.5, between A2 and A3 shades. The NW hue was created for whiter teeth (low Chroma and high value) and its two tabs were design to match adjacent bleached teeth.

The *Toothguide 3D-MASTER* shade guide (VITA Zahnfabrik), however, is shade guide already structured on Value (Fig. 3.7). The *Toothguide 3D-MASTER* shade guide is based on the principle of choosing color in three quick steps. First, selecting an appropriate value (from 1 to 5)

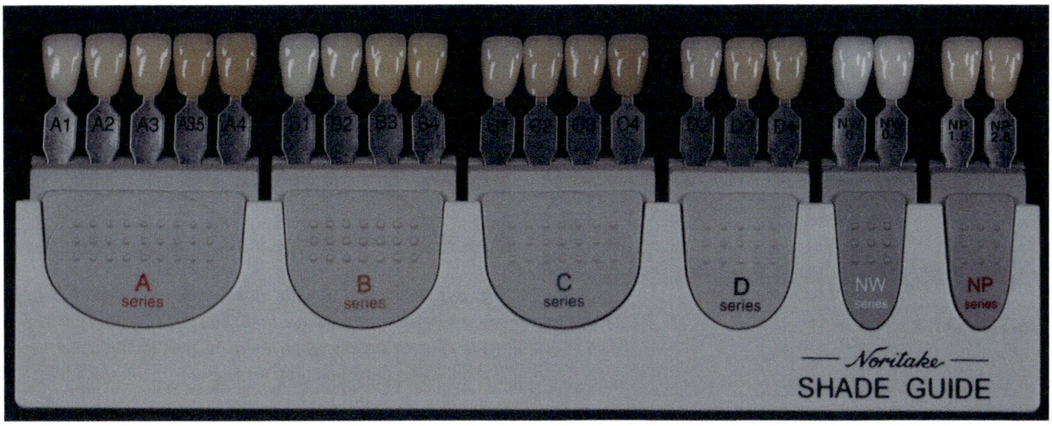

Fig. 3.6 Ceramic shade guides: *A–D* (Ivoclar Vivadent)

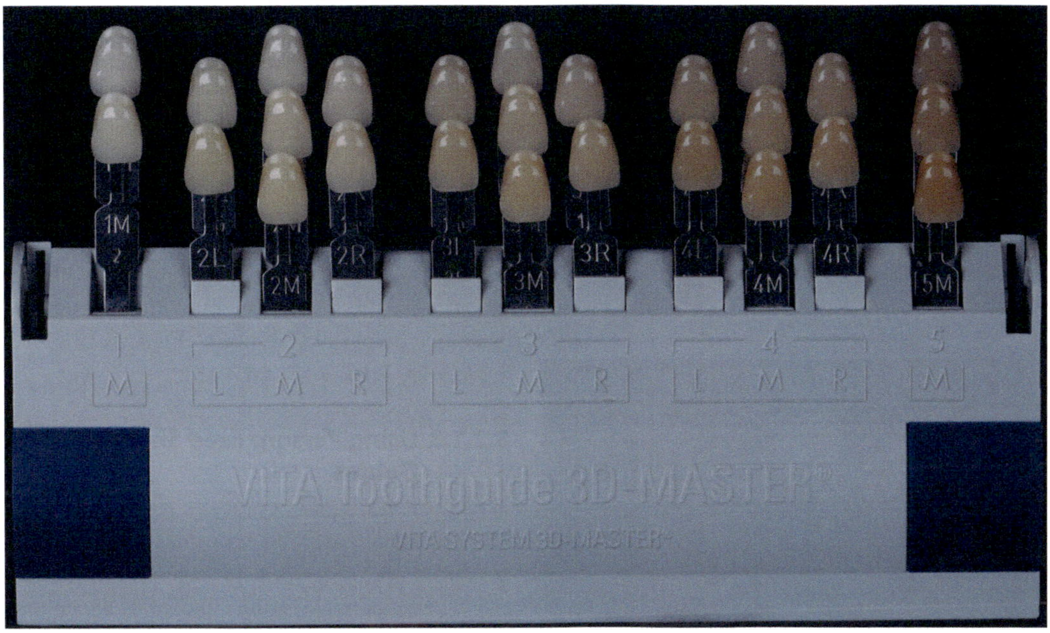

Fig. 3.7 Ceramic shade guides: *Toothguide 3D-MASTER* shade guide (VITA Zahnfabrik)

according to the patient's tooth. Then, selecting the corresponding Chroma into that value. In this step, it is recommended to choose the middle hue group (M) to determine the Chroma (from 1 up to 3). Finally, choosing the final color, checking whether the patient's tooth is more reddish (R) or more yellowish (L) in comparison to the guide tab. In order to simplify the color selection of *Toothguide 3D-MASTER*, the *Linearguide 3D-MASTER* shade guide (VITA Zahnfabrik), was introduced in 2008 (Figs. 3.8, 3.9, 3.10 and 3.11). It contains the same shade tabs but with simplified presentation and a two-step shade matching procedure: only 6 (step 1) and up to 7 (step 2) linearly arranged tabs instead of 29 tabs presented at the beginning of a three-step procedure with *Toothguide 3D-MASTER*.

3.2.1.2 Using Shade Guides for Composites

The majority of resin-based composites colors are named based on the *Vitapan Classical* color distribution concept. However, several other

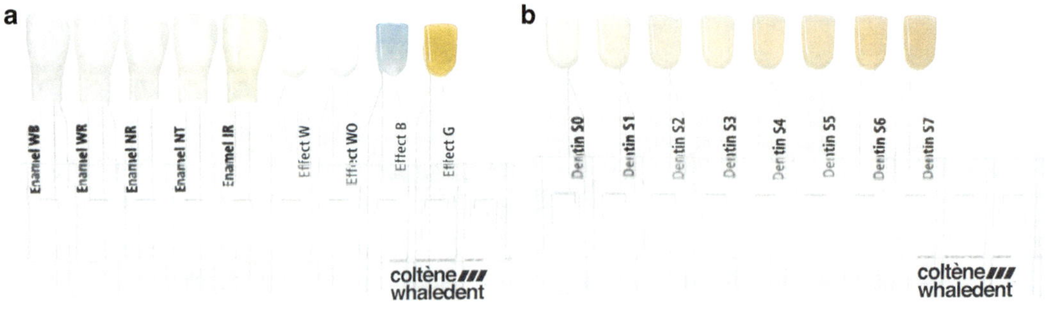

Fig. 3.14 (**a**) Composite shade guides: dentin shades of Miris2 system (Coltene). (*Photography courtesy of Coltene*). (**b**) Composite shade guides: enamel and effect shades of Miris2 system (Coltene). (*Photography courtesy of Coltene*)

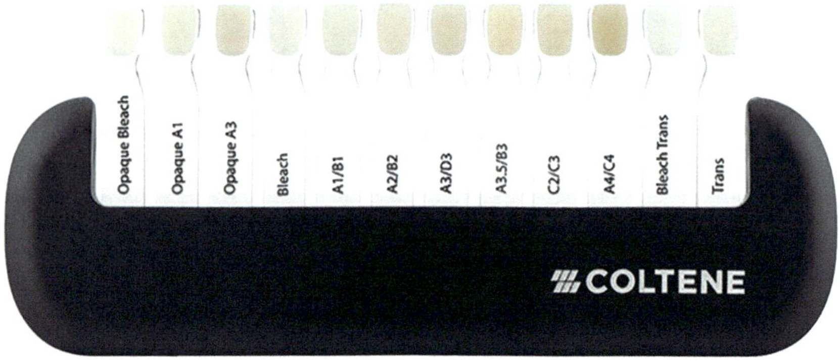

Fig. 3.15 Composite shade guide: Brillant system (Coltene). (*Photography courtesy of Coltene*)

Fig. 3.16 Composite shade guide: Opallis system (FGM)

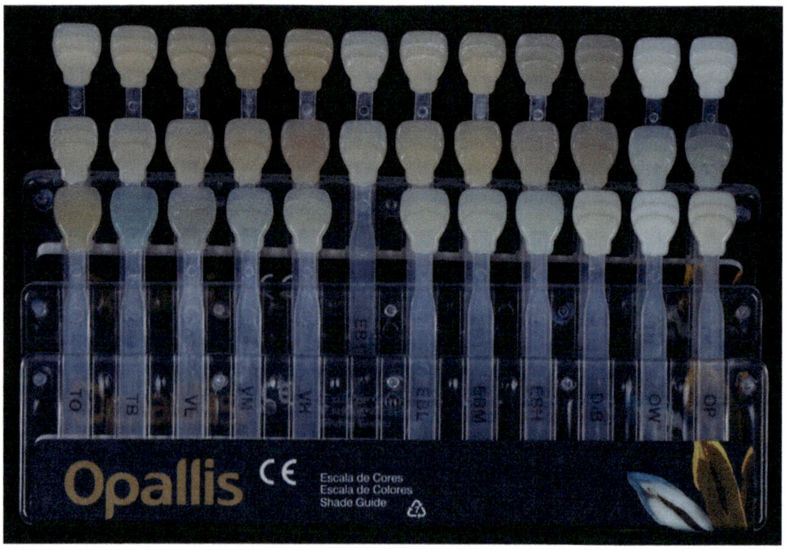

be registered as well as the respective color map draw (further explained in Chap. 7).

The resin composite that is not polymerized into the syringe is usually darker than the photopolymerized increment used during resin placement. These color differences are mainly caused by a decrease in lightness and Chroma after photopolymerization. In general, the decrease in lightness occurs because the monomers form polymers through the polymerization process. This reaction causes the reduction of their refractive indices, thus changing the way the light is transmitted, reflected, and refracted. The decrease in Chroma, however, occurs due to the consumption of the photoinitiator during the photoactivation process. Camphorquinone is the most commonly used photoinitiator in Dentistry. However, as a yellow-colored molecule, after reacting, its consumption leads to a decrease in composite yellowness.

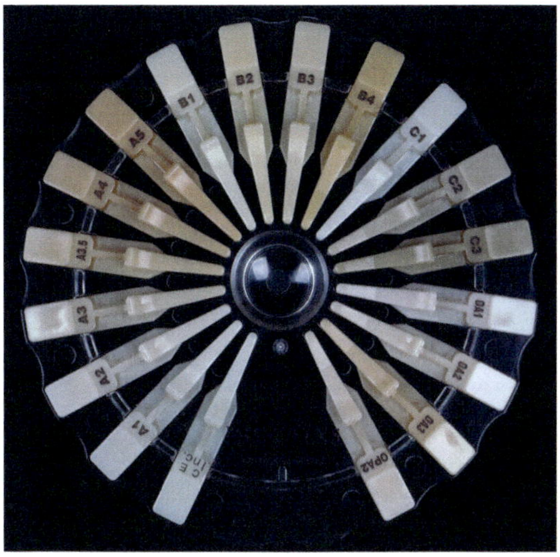

Fig. 3.17 Composite shade guide: Palfique system (Tokuyama)

3.2.1.5 Using the Mock-up Technique

To confirm the selected composite colors, regardless of shade selection technique (e.g., using ceramic or composite shade guide tabs or by increments of composites), a color mock-up may be made [7]. It is a non-bonded full shape restoration made free-handed. Then, it is flaked off from the tooth to observe the layering from both inner and outer aspects. It provides the opportunity to "rehearse" the contour and thickness of each den-

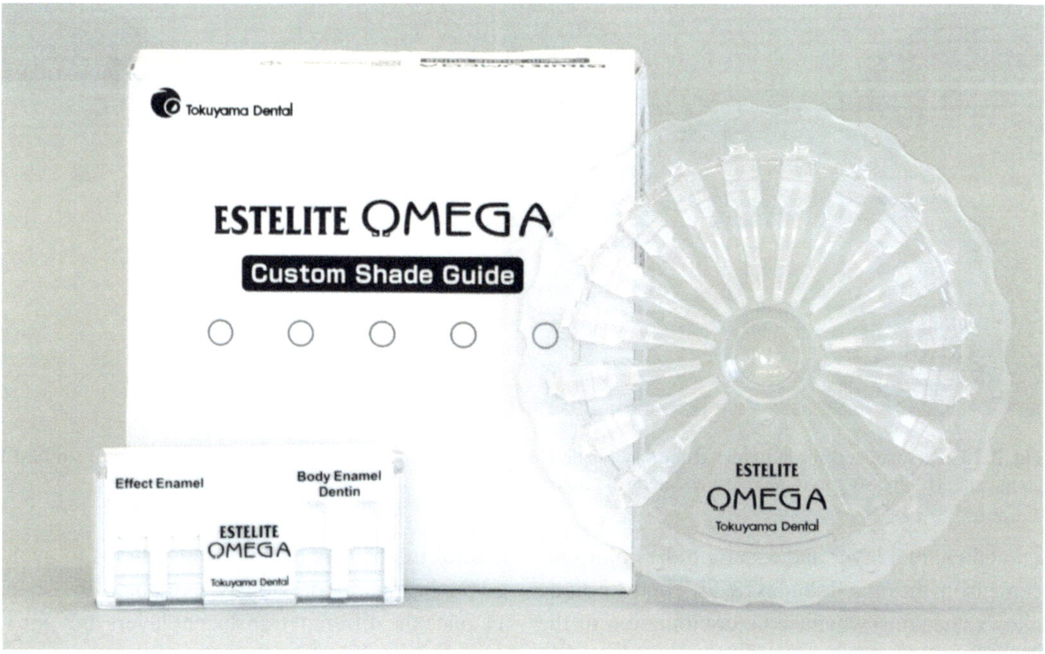

Fig. 3.18 Composite shade guide: Estelite Omega system (Tokuyama). (*Photography courtesy of Tokuyama Dental*)

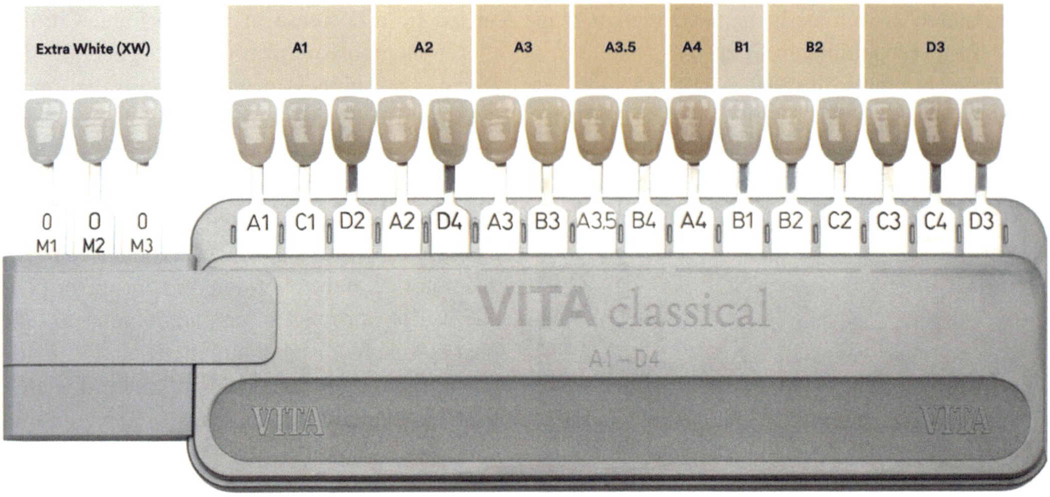

Fig. 3.19 Composite shade guide: Filtek Universal system (3M). (*Photography courtesy of 3M*)

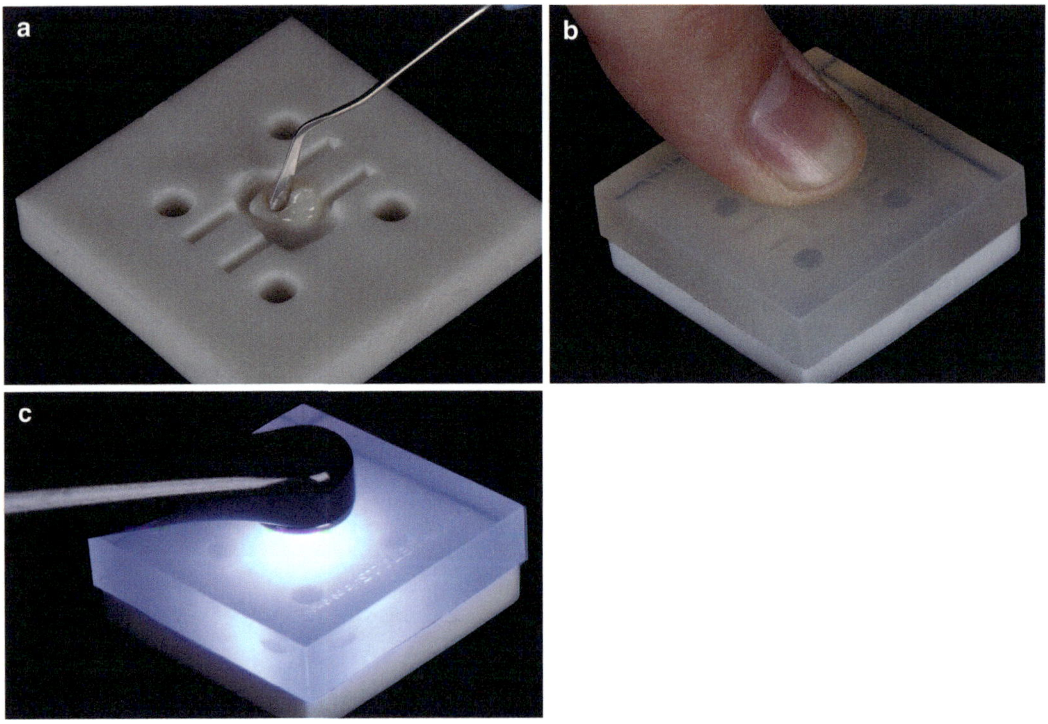

Fig. 3.20 Personalized shade guides using My Shade Guide (Smile Line): (**a**) filling a rubber mold with resin-based composite; (**b**) pressing to remove excess; and (**c**) photoactivation

tin and enamel layer and ascertain the color outcome from the mixed shades [8, 9]. This technique allows checking whether the combination of the different shades that were chosen to do really match with the polychromatic appearance of the natural tooth. This technique also helps to avoid goniochromism (previously explained in Chap. 1), once the different translucent layers are reproduced to confirm the final color of the restoration from different angles.

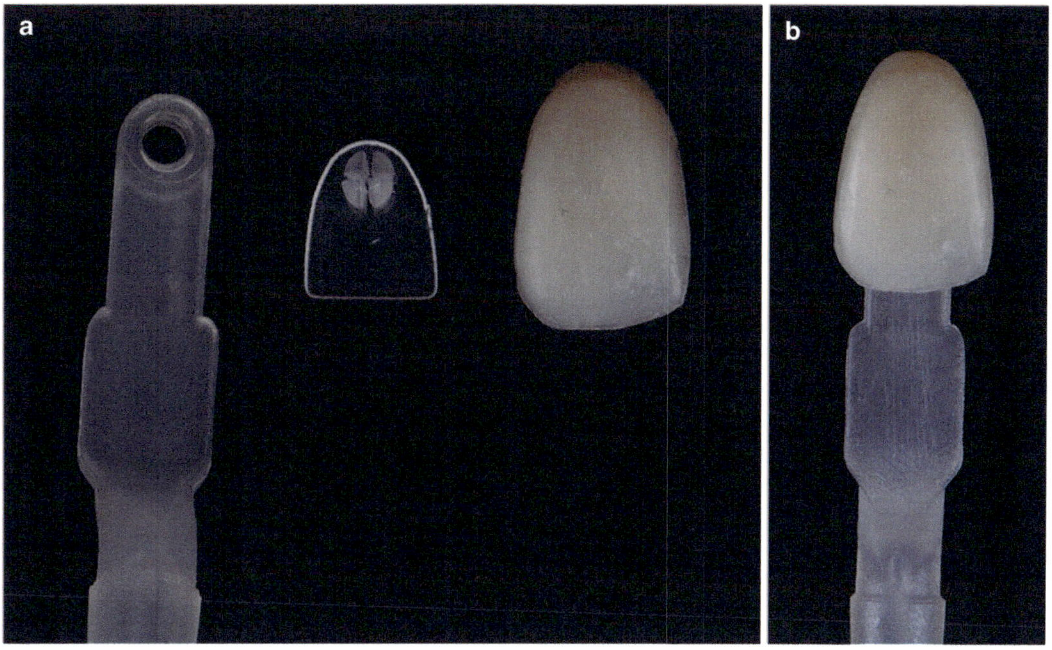

Fig. 3.21 Personalized shade guides using My Shade Guide (Smile Line): crafted tab of resin-based composite, before (**a**) and after (**b**) joining pieces

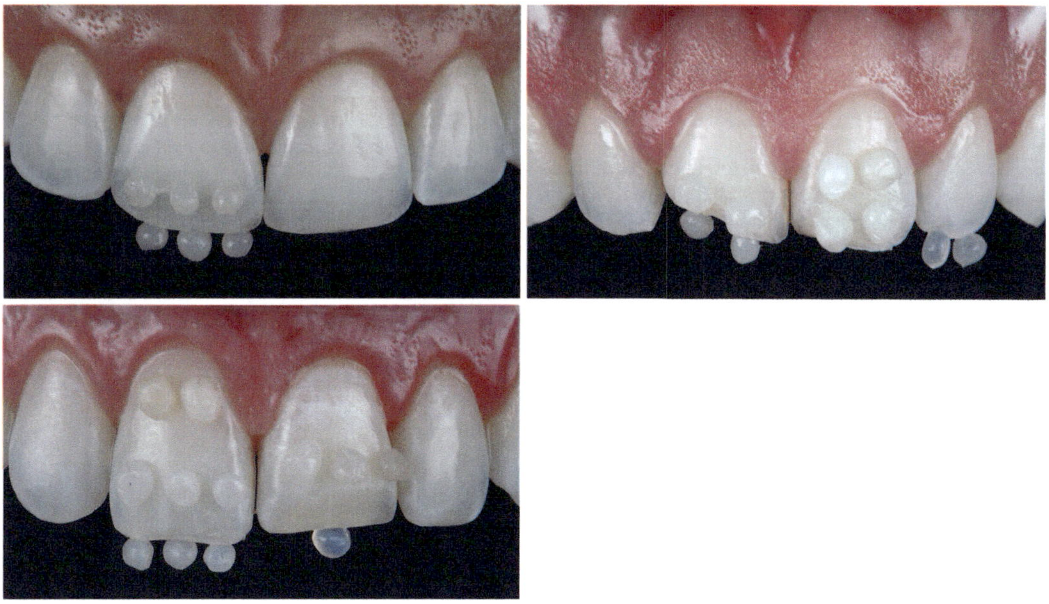

Figs. 3.22–3.24 Visual color selection for direct restorations using increments of composite according to different layering concepts

3.2.1.6 Visual Color Measurement Technique

Color from any object, as the tooth and shade guide tab, is directly influenced by illumination. Then, it is essential to place the tab equally leveled with teeth to get the same amount of illumination (Fig. 3.25). To perform an optimized color measurement, first, patients should be asked to remove any lipstick or shiny lip balms. The patient should be asked to sit and tilt his head up, pointing their smile towards the ceiling light. The shade guide must be brought close to the smile to initially pre-select a few coloring tabs.

Then, lip retractors should be used to expose teeth, and a black or gray background should be inserted behind them to neutralize the reddish influence of the oral cavity tissues (Figs. 3.26, 3.27, 3.28 and 3.29). Finally, one at a time, the pre-selected tabs should be mirrored placed close

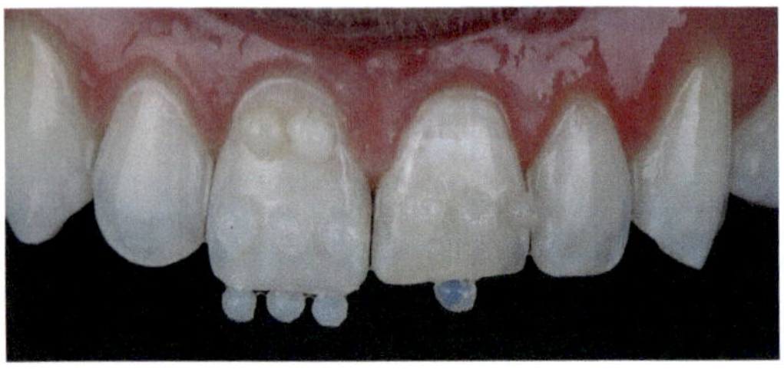

Fig. 3.25 Visual color selection for direct restorations using increments of composite: after photoactivation, teeth and restorative material should be wet for visual observation

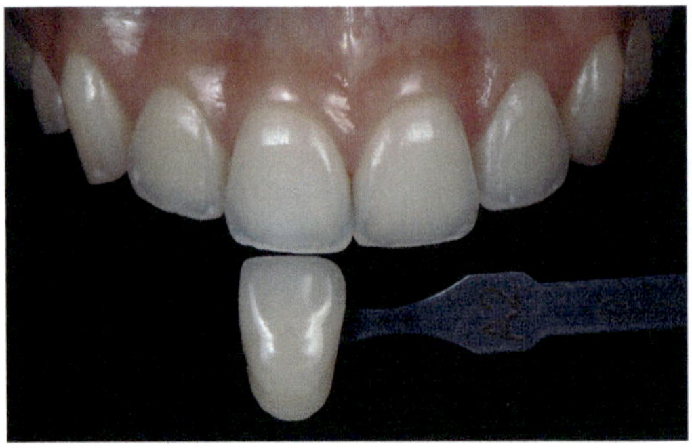

Fig. 3.26 Visual color selection for direct restorations using shade tabs: mirrored shade tab placement to teeth in order to get the same amount of illumination

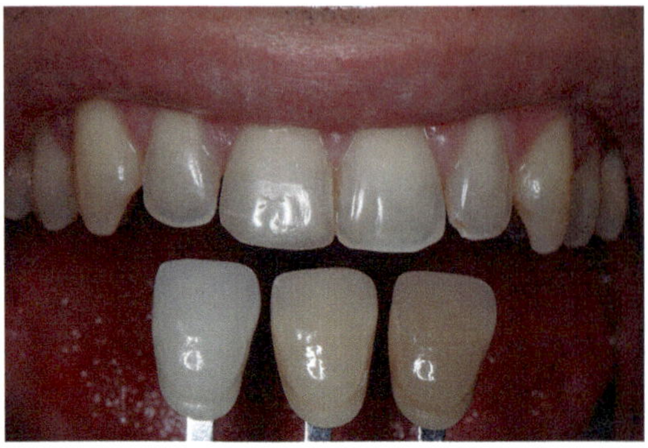

Fig. 3.27 Visual color selection for direct restorations using shade tabs: different shade tabs mirrored placed to teeth without any neutral background

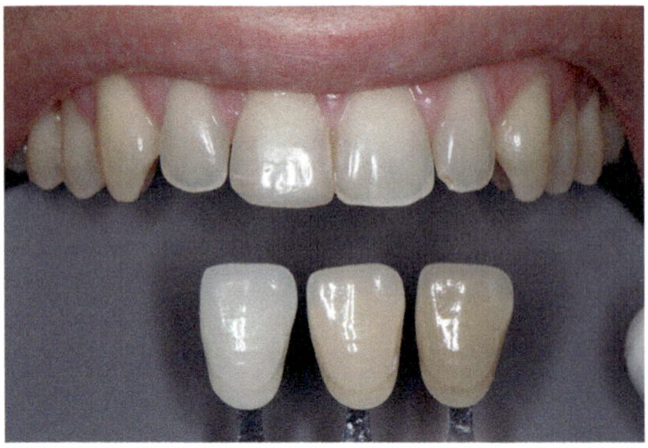

Fig. 3.28 Visual color selection for direct restorations using shade tabs: placement of a gray background behind upper teeth to neutralize the reddish influence of oral cavity background

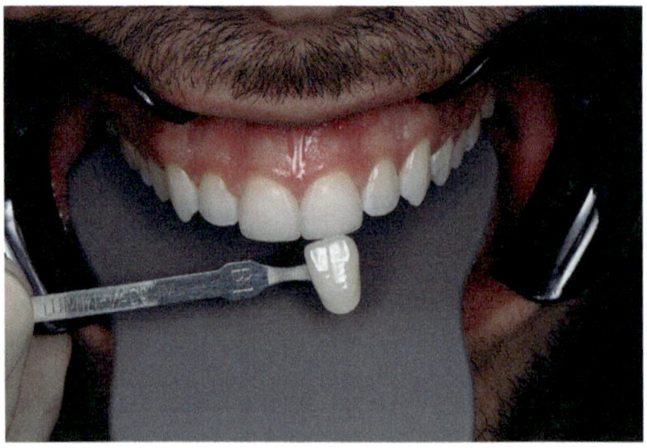

Fig. 3.29 Visual color selection for direct restorations using shade tabs: importance of lip retraction to provide proper illumination to teeth and shade tab

to the tooth to receive the same amount of light. Therefore, the tab that most closely matches the tooth color should be registered. Visual observation should not exceed 5 s to avoid color misinterpretation due to visual fatigue.

As previously described in Chap. 1, several factors can negatively influence the correct color measurement by visual methods, including variations in the type, quality, and intensity of light, professional's color blindness or deficiency in color perception, differences in gender and professional's experience [10–13].

Visual color measurements should be taken at ideal illumination conditions. As earlier explained in this chapter, a light source suitable for visual observation should have correlated color temperature of a full-spectrum balanced light between 5500 and 6500 K. During the visual shade matching, the light intensity should be diffuse, allowing clinicians to perceive color accurately and comfortably. The recommended lighting intensity for the dental office is 200–300 fc or 500–600 lx [2, 14]. Light-correcting devices are available to minimize the external lighting interference of dental offices due to variations in the daytime, the season of the year, and the resultant mixture between daylight and fluorescent or incandescent light from the room. Handheld light-emitting diode devices with 5500 K of color temperature can be used for this purpose as the *Rite-Lite* 2 and the *Rite-Lite Pro* (Addent) (previously illustrated, Figs. 3.2 and 3.3), and the *Smile Lite* and the *Smile Lite MPD* (Smile Line) (Figs. 3.30 and 3.31).

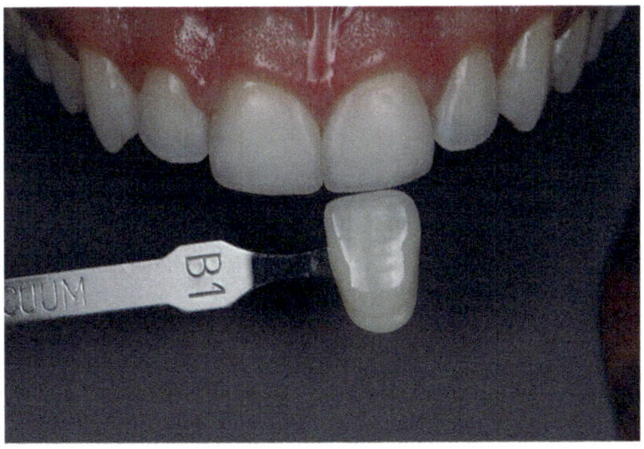

Fig. 3.30 Visual color selection for direct restorations using shade tabs: zoomed view of operative field in ideal lighting conditions

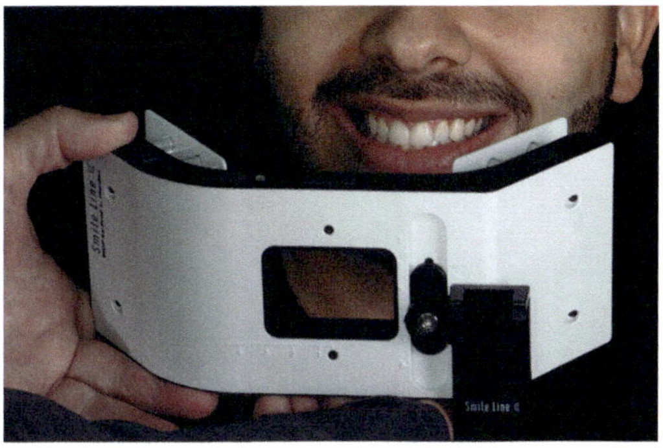

Fig. 3.31 Use of a portable light-correcting device to color measurement: *Smile Lite MPD* (Smile Line)

3.2.2 Objective Measurements

Clinically, the objective tooth color measurement can be assessed by different dental shade-matching devices that have been brought to the market to surpass the inconsistencies of visual shade matching. Examples are the spectrophotometers [15, 16] and the colorimeters [17, 18].

The dental spectrophotometers measure the amount of light energy reflected from the tooth surface at different wavelengths (1–25 nm intervals) of the visible spectrum and convert the numerical color values (CIELAB color coordinates) to the equivalent tab from a dental shade guide. *CrystalEye* (Olympus America), *Vita Easyshade V* (VITA), *Shade-X* (X-Rite), and *SpectroShade Micro* (MHT) are commercially available examples of dental spectrophotometers. On the other hand, dental colorimeters do not register spectral reflectance; they measure tooth color according to the tristimulus values (CIE XYZ) by filtering the reflected light into red, green, and blue areas of the visible spectrum and converting these to CIELAB color coordinates, and then to the correspondent tab from dental shade guide [19]. *ShadeVision* (X-Rite) is a commercially available example of a dental imaging colorimeter.

Colorimeters and spectrophotometers have broad application in tooth whitening longitudinal studies, and they can be used clinically to evaluate tooth color variation during the whitening treatment period. However, clinicians must take care to avoid inaccurate measurements when

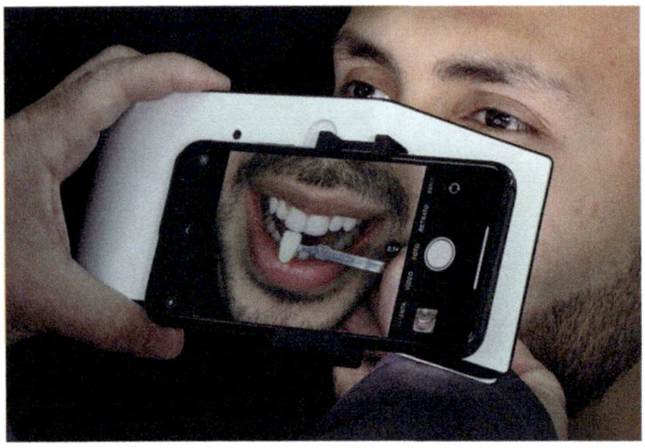

Fig. 3.32 Using a phone to register photographically the shade matching with the *Smile Lite MPD* (Smile Line)

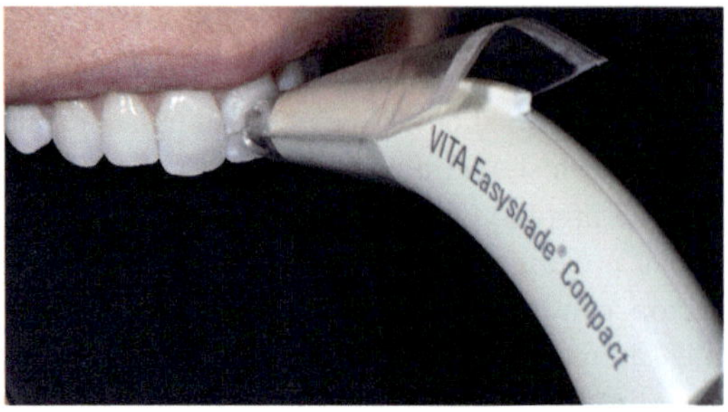

Fig. 3.33 Objective color measurement using Vita Easyshade V. (*Photography courtesy of Bryce Brandfon, Franciele Floriani, and Nathalie Sawczuk*)

using these devices. Since they are contact-measuring instruments, the results can be affected by the wrong positioning of the measuring probe, fogging of the optical lens, ambient illuminant used, and by the background, while taking the measurements [20, 21].

These devices have different prices, designs, software, and data output. They can measure the tooth's overall surface color or in limited areas. Overall tooth surface color measurement devices such as the *CrystaEye*, the *SpectroShade Micro*, and the *ShadeVision* provide a color map with the correspondent color tab from a shade guide according to the tooth three thirds: cervical, body, and incisal. Limited area measurement devices such as the *Easyshade V*, and the *Shade-X* provide the color correspondent the color tab from a shade guide according to the 3–5 mm diameter area of measurement of the tip of the probe of the device. For this reason, to monitor color change during tooth whitening, for example, the probe should be placed in the center of the middle third from the tooth buccal surface (Fig. 3.32).

The tooth color can also be objectively measured by image analysis techniques obtained with digital cameras [22–24] or intraoral digital scanners [25–27]. Despite the encouragement of its use to improve communication with dental technicians to diminish the color matching disagreement among teeth and indirect restorations, and even their indication for research studies, its clinical use to monitor color change during tooth whitening treatments is still a challenge due to its complexity (Fig. 3.33).

References

1. Clary JA, Ontiveros JC, Cron SG, Paravina RD. Influence of light source, polarization, education and training on shade matching quality. J Prosthet Dent. 2016;116(1):91–7.
2. Gasparik C, Grecu AG, Culic B, Badea ME, Dudea D. Shade-matching performance using a new light-correcting device. J Esthet Restor Dent. 2015;27(5):285–92.
3. Joiner A. Tooth colour: a review of the literature. J Dent. 2004;32(Suppl 1):3–12.
4. Browning WD, Contreras-Bulnes R, Brackett MG, Brackett WW. Color differences: polymerized composite and corresponding Vitapan classical shade tab. J Dent. 2009;37(Suppl 1):e34–9.
5. Fahl N Jr. Single-shaded direct anterior composite restorations: a simplified technique for enhanced results. Compend Contin Educ Dent. 2012;33(2):150–4.
6. Dietschi D, Fahl N Jr. Shading concepts and layering techniques to master direct anterior composite restorations: an update. Br Dent J. 2016;221(12):765–71.
7. Dietschi D. Free-hand bonding in the esthetic treatment of anterior teeth: creating the illusion. J Esthet Dent. 1997;9(4):156–64.
8. Fahl N Jr. Achieving ultimate anterior esthetics with a new microhybrid composite. Compend Contin Educ Dent Suppl. 2000;26:4–13.
9. Dietschi D. Optimising aesthetics and facilitating clinical application of free-hand bonding using the 'natural layering concept'. Br Dent J. 2008;204(4):181–5.

10. Della Bona A, Barrett AA, Rosa V, Pinzetta C. Visual and instrumental agreement in dental shade selection: three distinct observer populations and shade matching protocols. Dent Mater. 2009;25(2):276–81.
11. Simionato A, Pecho OE, Della BA. Efficacy of color discrimination tests used in dentistry. J Esthet Restor Dent. 2020;33(6):865–73.
12. Pecho OE, Ghinea R, Perez MM, Della BA. Influence of gender on visual shade matching in dentistry. J Esthet Restor Dent. 2017;29(2):E15–23.
13. Samra APB, Moro MG, Mazur RF, Vieira S, De Souza EM, Freire A, Rached RN. Performance of dental students in shade matching: impact of training. J Esthet Restor Dent. 2017;29(2):E24–32.
14. Wee AG, Meyer A, Wu W, Wichman CS. Lighting conditions used during visual shade matching in private dental offices. J Prosthet Dent. 2016;115(4):469–74.
15. Chen H, Huang J, Dong X, Qian J, He J, Qu X, Lu E. A systematic review of visual and instrumental measurements for tooth shade matching. Quintessence Int. 2012;43(8):649–59.
16. Kim-Pusateri S, Brewer JD, Davis EL, Wee AG. Reliability and accuracy of four dental shade-matching devices. J Prosthet Dent. 2009;101(3):193–9.
17. Li Q, Wang YN. Comparison of shade matching by visual observation and an intraoral dental colorimeter. J Oral Rehabil. 2007;34(11):848–54.
18. Karaagaclioglu L, Terzioglu H, Yilmaz B, Yurdukoru B. In vivo and in vitro assessment of an intraoral dental colorimeter. J Prosthodont. 2010;19(4):279–85.
19. Chu SJ, Trushkowsky RD, Paravina RD. Dental color matching instruments and systems. Review of clinical and research aspects. J Dent. 2010;38(Suppl 2):e2–16.
20. Chu SJ. Use of a reflectance spectrophotometer in evaluating shade change resulting from tooth-whitening products. J Esthet Restor Dent. 2003;15(s1):S42–8.
21. Raoufi S, Birkhed D. Effect of whitening toothpastes on tooth staining using two different colour-measuring devices—a 12-week clinical trial. Int Dent J. 2010;60(6):419–23.
22. Gerlach RW, Barker ML, Sagel PA. Objective and subjective whitening response of two self-directed bleaching systems. Am J Dent. 2002;15:7A–12A.
23. Wee AG, Lindsey DT, Kuo S, Johnston WM. Color accuracy of commercial digital cameras for use in dentistry. Dent Mater. 2006;22(6):553–9.
24. Lasserre JF, Pop-Ciutrila IS, Colosi HA. A comparison between a new visual method of colour matching by intraoral camera and conventional visual and spectrometric methods. J Dent. 2011;39(Suppl 3):e29–36.
25. Liberato WF, Barreto IC, Costa PP, Almeida CC, Pimentel W, Tiossi R. A comparison between visual, intraoral scanner, and spectrophotometer shade matching: a clinical study. J Prosthet Dent. 2019;121(2):271–5.
26. Yoon HI, Bae JW, Park JM, Chun YS, Kim MA, Kim M. A study on possibility of clinical application for color measurements of shade guides using an intraoral digital scanner. J Prosthodont. 2018;27(7):670–5.
27. Ebeid K, Sabet A, Della BA. Accuracy and repeatability of different intraoral scanners on shade determination. J Esthet Restor Dent. 2020;33(6):844–8.

4 Color Evaluation for Research Purposes

Camila Sampaio and Pablo Atria

4.1 Introduction

According to published surveys, color education, color training, and shade matching programs are receiving increased attention over the last decade, according to published surveys [1]. This fact is directly related to patients' expectations and demands in achieving dental restorations that can mirror their adjacent natural teeth or improve their tooth esthetical characteristics with colored artificial restorations [2]. In this topic, color can be underrated, as patients do not often explicitly ask for the "color of their restorations." Instead, they expect functional, long-lasting, and esthetic restorations, with color being put as a background, unimportant or taken for granted, even though it could be the decisive factor in the overall acceptance of the treatment itself [3].

A few years from now, color was not such a trendy and studied topic, but today it is considered an ever-expanding field, equally relevant for clinical application, research, and education [4]. Due to advances in color measurement, digital instruments can promote a numerical measurement, allowing color to be metrically recorded and evaluated, which favored color matching, communication, reproduction, and verification in clinical and research dentistry. This approach was changed back in 1973 and 1974 when Sproul stated that "the technology of color is not a simple matter that can be learned without study; neither is it a complicated matter beyond dentists' comprehension" [5]. After that, a huge effort was put on new teaching methods using modern technology to help dental professionals and dental students to learn about color in an organized and comprehensive manner. Nowadays, scientific journals have editorials whose objective is specifically to study color and its influences on shade matching and color changes [2].

Color is defined as the result of the interaction of light with an object, which means that a given object's compositional characteristics greatly impact the way light is absorbed by or reflected from this object, as further explained in Chap. 1 [6]. The natural teeth are polychromatic, meaning many colors and optical characteristics can be perceived when observed under ideal light conditions [6]. Since enamel, dentin, and pulp present different composition, they also interact with light differently, resulting in an extremely complex interaction, which is difficult to be reproduced with artificial materials [6]. Differences between younger and older teeth exist regarding the color value, Chroma, and transparency. For instance, young teeth present a high color value due to the high quantity of enamel, while older

C. Sampaio (✉)
College of Dentistry, University of the Andes, Santiago, Chile
e-mail: CSampaio@miuandes.cl

P. Atria
Biomedical Engineering, New York University, New York, NY, USA

D. Oliveira (ed.), *Color Science and Shade Selection in Operative Dentistry*,
https://doi.org/10.1007/978-3-030-99173-9_4

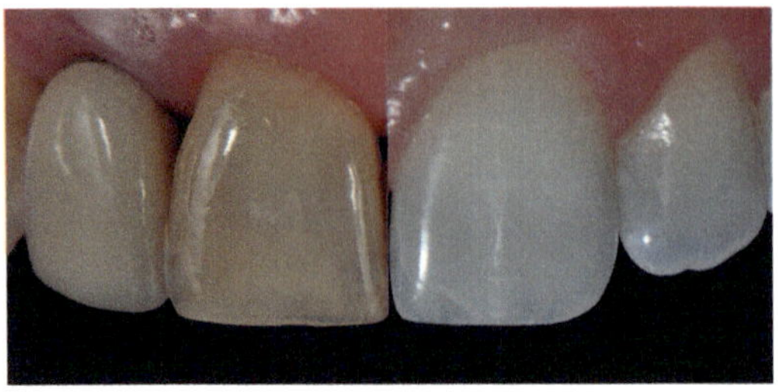

Fig. 4.1 Color and texture comparison of older (left) and younger (right) teeth. Observe the lower color value present on the older teeth, while a higher color value is observed in the younger teeth. Moreover, some regions of the older teeth can be observed as almost transparent due to the thickness of the substrate, while in the younger teeth, the original teeth textures and translucencies can be noted

teeth present a much lower color value than that which is seen in younger teeth, as it becomes thinner and more translucent over time, sometimes becoming nearly transparent (Fig. 4.1) [7].

4.2 Visual Methods to Evaluate Color

Color is defined as a combination of hue, Chroma, and value. Hue is defined as the name of color itself, for instance, red or yellow. Chroma is the degree of hue saturation, or the intensity exhibited by a color. Finally, value is defined as the brightness or luminosity of color [8]. Although no single method is considered standard, two methods exist to evaluate color in dentistry, which are visual and instrumental. Several kinds of research compare both methods revealing their pros and cons. One important finding of such research is that both methods should be used together whenever it is possible, as they can complement each other and lead to a predictable esthetic outcome [9].

The visual method is often considered subjective, as it can exhibit a higher level of inconsistencies for both intra-rater and inter-rater comparisons, while instrumental or digital methods can exhibit significantly higher reliability [10]; also, it is strongly dependent on the interaction between light and the dental structure. However, it is also the most common method used in dental practice and should not be underrated.

Visual methods consist of the observer visually selecting the best match for an object when this object is compared visually to tooth color examples such as shade guides. The shade guides most commonly used in the dental practice, as well as in research, are the VITA Classical shade guide and the VITA Toothguide 3D-Master System, both from VITA Zahnfabrik (Bad Säckingen, Germany) [1]. The Vitapan Classical shade guide configuration is also known as A-to-D arrangement, divided into 16 tabs originally arranged into four groups based on hue and within the groups according to increasing Chroma [11]. On the other hand, the Vitapan 3-D Master shade tabs are arranged three-dimensionally, divided into groups according to lightness, and within the groups according to saturation (vertically) and hue (horizontally) [12]. Six different levels of lightness were used to create six groups of tabs, from 0 (the lightest) to 5 (the darkest). There are 3 Chroma levels, from 1 (the least chromatic) to 3 (the most chromatic) in each group (except in group 1 that has two Chroma levels). Intermediate Chroma levels (1.5 and 2.5) in groups 2, 3, and 4 are associated with hue variations—L (less red) and R (more red). More recently, the same brand launched the Linearguide 3D-Master [11]. Other brands also have their A–D arrangements shade guides, which can correlate (although not 100% accurately) to the Vitapan Classical shade guide [13].

With this being said, when performing visual selection, the final color decision is totally operator-dependent. Studies demonstrated that the color preferences of observers and shade selection are dependent on: the level of experience of the operator, with education and training presenting a statistically significant improvement in shade matching [3, 14]; the operator's gender, with some studies showing that females are better in color match than males [15, 16], while other indicates that this is not a decisive factor [15, 17];

on the type of color, with darker and more chromatic shade tabs being more often mismatched [3, 17]; on skin shades and gingival shades, among others [18, 19].

Increased shade matching accuracy can be translated into enhanced dental restorations esthetics, increased patient satisfaction, and reduced color corrections [3]. For that purpose, manufacturers are launching restorative materials with visual color adjustment potential to blend with the surrounding enamel and dentin, resulting in reduced color differences and, therefore, improving the restoration's esthetic appearance, simplifying the shade matching compensating for any color mismatch [9, 20].

When performing visual shade matching only, the only color information provided to the technician by many clinicians is the laboratory prescription. However, a method to improve shade matching with this technique is by performing a color map (Fig. 4.2), which can be simply drawn in the lab prescription or sent in a photograph. A simple photograph taken with a smartphone can be manipulated and improves shade matching and decreasing color difference values (ΔE) of the comparison between the restoration performed by the technician and the tooth color of comparison, as observed in a recent study [21]. This subject will be discussed below and can help in achieving a more accurate shade selection result.

4.2.1 Color Blindness Test or Ishihara Test

Color blindness, color deficiency, or color vision alteration occur when the correct determination of the color of an object is altered. It is presented in about 8% of the male population and 0.5% of the female population [22]. This alteration affects the ability to identify the red, green, yellow, or blue colors in charge of cells located in the retina called cones. On the other hand, detecting changes in value or luminosity is not influenced by color deficiencies. It depends on retinal circuits other than photoreceptor cells [22]. When testing for color blinding, graphic designs and illustrations can be created and used, with tests consisting of numbered colored plates, mostly known as Ishihara plates containing a circle of dots appearing randomized in color and size (Fig. 4.3).

In research, except for the studies which have as main objective evaluating people with color deficiencies [22], studies on color training typically exclude those individuals [17–19, 23, 24]. However, many times color deficiencies are an

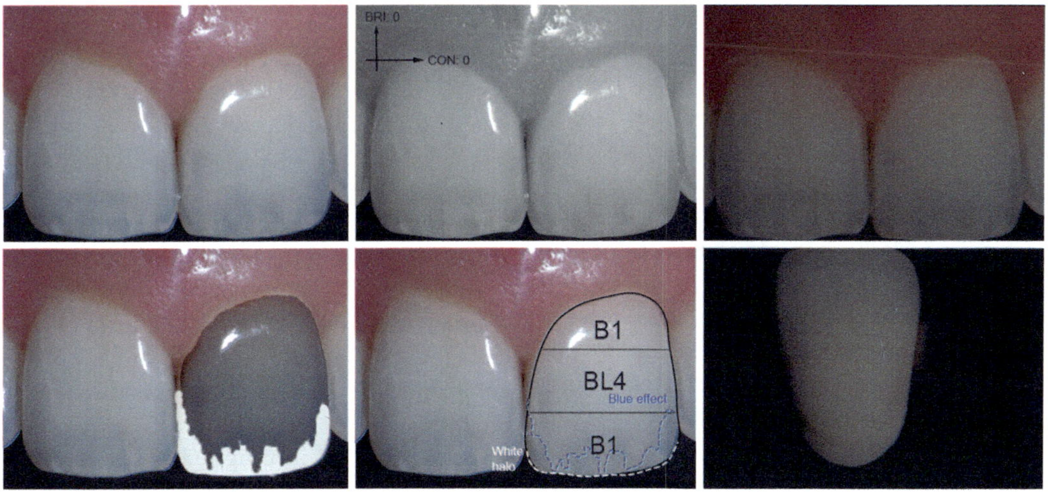

Fig. 4.2 Example of Ishihara vision testing chart

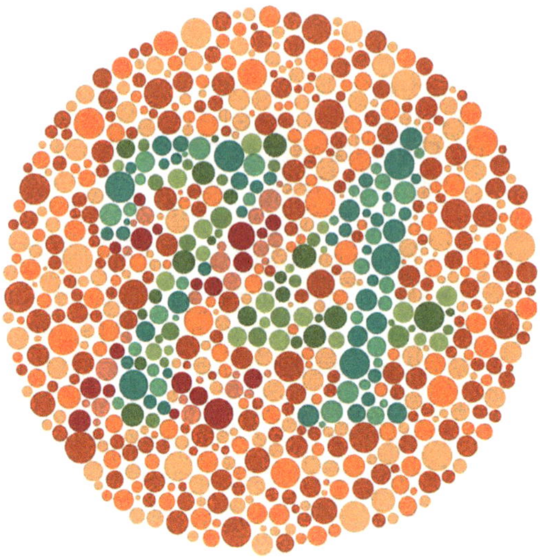

Fig. 4.3 Color mapping of teeth, important information can be reported to lab technicians with color maps, this can be done drawn in a lab prescription or in photographic means, through digital cameras or smartphones, which allow color manipulation by both dentist and technician

underdiagnosed disease, but very relevant in people who study Dentistry.

Participants for research purposes are usually screened or tested for their color vision, participating in an evaluation of perceptibility and visual acceptability judgments in Dentistry [24], and need to pass a dental color matching competency, according to the ISO/TR 28642:2016 [25]. For example, participants need to match at least 60% of the pairs of tabs from Vita Classical shade guide (below 60%—no competency). Minimum of 60% (10 pairs of tabs), 75% (12 pairs), and 85% (14 pairs) corresponded to poor, average, and superior color matching competency, respectively [20]. A previous study concluded that observers with superior color matching competence could achieve better color matching results than those with the average color discrimination competence [17].

It is important to point out that the human eye is more sensitive to changes in luminosity and less sensitive to changes in tone. Every person should perceive changes in the value before perceiving changes in the hue Chroma of a tooth [26]. Value is a fundamental aspect that must be established successfully to correct color in esthetic restorations [26, 27].

4.2.2 Color Perception × Color Acceptance Thresholds

A visual threshold consists of perceiving a difference in color and whether this difference is visually acceptable or not, or in other words, which are recognizable and tolerable. Color thresholds are important not only in the field of Dentistry, but also serve as quality control for a number of applications [4]. It also helps evaluating the clinical performance of materials, both in the clinical practice and in vivo and in vitro research, evaluating and interpreting a clinical outcome, and standardization. The importance of quality control in dentistry is reinforced by increased patients' and dental professionals' esthetic demands [4].

When performing color thresholds, the color perception threshold question is: "Can you see a difference in color between these two specimens?" If the observer answered "yes" to this question, they were asked the acceptability threshold question: "Would you consider this difference to be color acceptable in a patient's mouth?" The psychometric function is then simply the percentage of "yes" responses as a function of specimen color difference; 50% "yes" responses were considered the threshold level [24]. Basically, this can be resumed as: when the color difference between compared objects can be seen by 50% of observers (the other 50% will notice no difference), we are talking about the 50:50 perceptibility threshold. When the color difference is considered acceptable by 50% of observers (the other 50% would consider it unacceptable), this corresponds to the 50:50 acceptability threshold. A color match in dentistry is a color difference at or below the former threshold; an acceptable color match is a color difference at or below the later one [28, 29].

Paravina et al. investigated the relationship between "50:50% perceptibility thresholds" and

"50:50% acceptability thresholds." They defined the terms "50:50% perceptibility threshold" or "50:50% acceptability threshold" and referred to values where 50% of the observers perceive, or still accept, respectively, a color difference. They found differences in shade selection of 50:50% perceptibility ($\Delta E_{ab} = 1.2$, $\Delta E_{00} = 0.8$) and 50:50% acceptability ($\Delta E_{ab} = 2.7$, $\Delta E_{00} = 1.8$) were significantly different [4]. These results were later implemented in the ISO 28642:2016 [25].

Although obviously, color matches at or below the perceptible threshold would be ideal, achieving a non-perceivable match is costly, time-consuming, and frequently not essential on a clinical basis [4]. The color difference formulas are important to allow a better correlation between visual judgments (perceptibility and acceptability) and instrumental color difference values [30].

4.3 Digital Methods to Evaluate Color

Instrumental methods have been used to improve color selection and communication and have been reported to be more reliable than the visual method used by itself. They became very popular in dental research due to the development of new technologies that are user-friendly and offer objective information on color specification, as well as magnitude and direction of color differences [31]. Dental shade matching instruments can overcome or reduce imperfections and inconsistencies of traditional shade matching with shade guides [28]. However, whenever possible, visual and instrumental methods should be combined [9], as it should not be forgotten that patient's visual judgment on color match or mismatch is usually the final and decisive one [31]. Advances in color measuring devices may remove a certain degree the subjectivity of the color determination and enhance the reliability of shade matching and shade communication [10]. Also, reliability is significantly better with the instrumental shade matching method than the visual method [10].

4.3.1 CIE-Lab and CIE-LCh

The CIE (Commission Internationale de l'Eclairage) has been traditionally involved in colorimetry for dental materials. It has been responsible for introducing the main color systems, illumination patterns, and color difference (ΔE) concepts used in color science [32]. In order to unify criteria about color and to simplify communication between professionals, the CIE developed the CIE-Lab system. With this system, all colors can be easily captured and described. The CIE-Lab color space system (Fig. 4.4) consists of describing the colors within the Cartesian coordinates as L, a^*, and b^*, where L^* is the lightness coordinate (brightness or value), which connects an imaginary south pole (0—black) with an imaginary north pole (100—white), and all gray values are represented in this vertical line. On the sphere's equator, all other saturated colors are shown, corresponding to the Chroma of the colors. The right angles in the equator plane, the a^*- and b^*-axis, that represent the directions of the color valences red–green (positive–negative) and yellow–blue (positive–negative), respectively. Each color has a specific numerical value, thus providing a more objective characterization and assisting in color communication [27].

In research, most of the studies quantify color differences using the CIE-Lab color space and associating with the ΔE, which is related to a color difference formula.

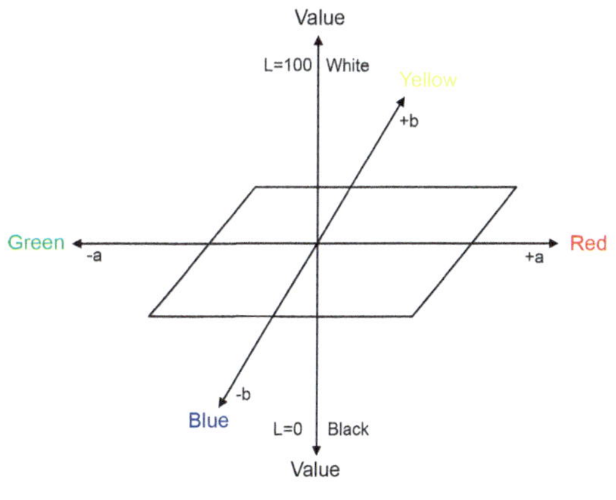

Fig. 4.4 CIE-Lab color space

When working with the CIE-LCh system and for more clearness, the Cartesian coordinates (L, a^*, b^*) can be converted into cylinder coordinates L, C, h° according to the following formulas:

$$C = \sqrt{a^2 + b^2}$$

$$h^\circ = \arctan\left(\frac{b}{a}\right),$$

where L remains unchanged, C (Chroma) represents the distance from the polar axis and represents the color intensity; and h° is the hue angle in the equatorial plane (Fig. 4.5). Hue angle starts at the $+a^*$ axis and is expressed in degrees (e.g., 0° is $+a^*$, or red, and 90° is $+b$, or yellow). It has the same diagram as the $L^*a^*b^*$ color space but uses cylindrical coordinates instead of rectangular coordinates [23].

4.3.2 Color Difference Formulas (ΔE)

Color difference formulas provide a quantitative representation of the perceived color difference (ΔE) between a pair of colored samples under a given set of experimental conditions [29]. Color difference has been used extensively in dental research and applications [30]. In the majority of dental color studies, color and color differences are quantified using the CIE-Lab color space and the associated ΔE_{ab}.

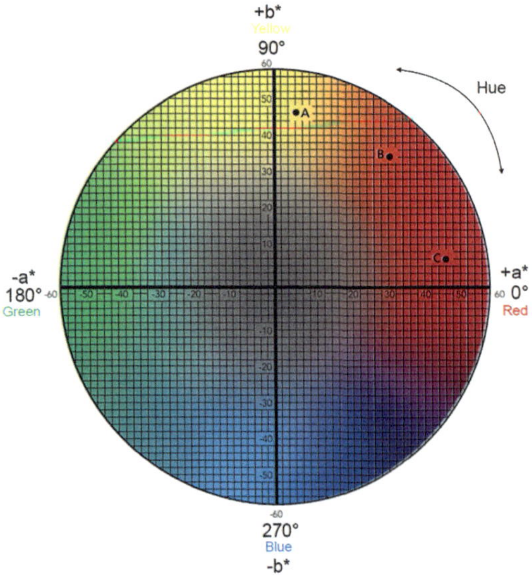

Fig. 4.5 CIE-LCh color space

- CIE76

  Based on the $L\ a^*b^*$ values of each color, color determination differences can be measured and evaluated. The $L\ a^*b^*$—or CIE-Lab color space (CIE of 1976) was the first formula to measure color difference (ΔE) according to the CIE-Lab coordinates. It is the most commonly used in publications and color differences (ΔE_{ab}) and is calculated according to the Euclidean difference formula [23]:

$$\Delta E_{ab} = \sqrt{(L1 - L2)^2 + (a1 - a2)^2 + (b1 - b2)^2}$$

$$\Delta E_{ab} = \sqrt{\Delta L^2 + \Delta a^2 + \Delta b^2}.$$

- CIE94

  The CIE94 formula is defined in the $L^*C^*h^*$ color space, showing the color differences in lightness (or value), Chroma and hue calculated from the Lab coordinates:

$$\Delta E_{*94} = \sqrt{\left(\frac{\Delta L_*}{K_L S_L}\right)^2 + \left(\frac{\Delta C^*_{ab}}{K_C S_C}\right)^2 + \left(\frac{\Delta H^*_{ab}}{K_H S_H}\right)^2}$$

$$\Delta L_* = L_1^* - L_2^*$$

$$C_1^* = \sqrt{a^{*\,2}_{\;1} + b^{*\,2}_{\;1}}.$$

- CIEDE2000

  Different color difference formulas were launched aiming to improve the correction between computed and perceived color differences and reflect the individual subjective impression of a color difference. Nowadays, the CIEDE2000 (ΔE_{00}) is the most accepted and CIE recommended color difference formula in dentistry, providing a better fit than the previous formulas, and therefore replacing them [30]. The CIEDE2000 utilizes the concepts of Chroma and hue, reinforcing the importance of the conceptual developments of Munsell [32]:

$$\Delta E_{*_{100}} = \sqrt{\left(\frac{\Delta L'}{K_L S_L}\right)^2 + \left(\frac{\Delta C'}{K_C S_C}\right)^2 + \left(\frac{\Delta H'}{K_H S_H}\right)^2 + R_T \frac{\Delta C'}{K_C S_C}\frac{\Delta H'}{K_H S_H}}.$$

It incorporates specific corrections for non-uniformity of CIE-Lab color space (the weighting functions: S_L, S_C, S_H), a rotation term (R_T) that accounts for the interaction between Chroma and hue differences in the blue region and a modification of the a^* coordinate of CIE-Lab, that mainly affects colors with low Chroma (neutral colors) and parameters accounting for the influence of illuminating and vision conditions in color difference evaluation (the parametric factors: K_L, K_C, K_H). The parametric factor ratio was proposed as a way to control changes in the magnitude of tolerance judgments and as a way to adjust for scaling of acceptability rather than perceptibility. Studies on visual judgments performed in textile color acceptability and dental ceramics acceptability showed that using $K_L = 2$ resulted in color differences better correlated to observations from a subset of average observers.

When compared, changes in color calculated with the CIE-LAB and the CIEDE2000 formulas followed similar trends but with different absolute values when calculated [33].

4.3.3 Spectrophotometers and Colorimeters

Spectrophotometers and colorimeters are among the most used instrumental shade matching methods in Dentistry and can be used to help overcome some shortcomings of a visual method by bringing accuracy and helping with shade matching, communication, and reproduction. Moreover, color measuring instruments can be valuable in shade verification (quality control) [19].

Spectrophotometers are among the most accurate, useful, and flexible instruments for overall color matching and color matching in dentistry [34]. They can measure the amount of light energy reflected from an object at 1–25 nm intervals along the visible spectrum [35, 36]. A spectrophotometer contains a source of optical radiation, a means of dispersing light, an optical system for measuring, a detector, and converting light obtained to a signal that can be analyzed. After that, the data obtained from spectrophotometers must be manipulated and translated into a form useful for dental professionals [28]. The instruments' measurements are frequently keyed to dental shade guides and converted to a shade tab equivalent [37]. Compared with observations by the human eye or conventional techniques, it was found that spectrophotometers offered a 33% increase in accuracy and a more objective match in 93.3% of the cases [38].

The most used and known spectrophotometer available in the market, used for both research and clinical aims, is the Vita Easyshade (Vita Zahnfabrik) (Fig. 4.6). It is a contact-type spectrophotometer that provides enough shade information to help aid in the color analysis process. Different measurement modes are possible with this instrument: tooth single-mode, tooth area mode (cervical, middle and incisal shades), restoration color verification (includes lightness, Chroma, and hue comparison), and shade tab mode (practice/training mode) [39].

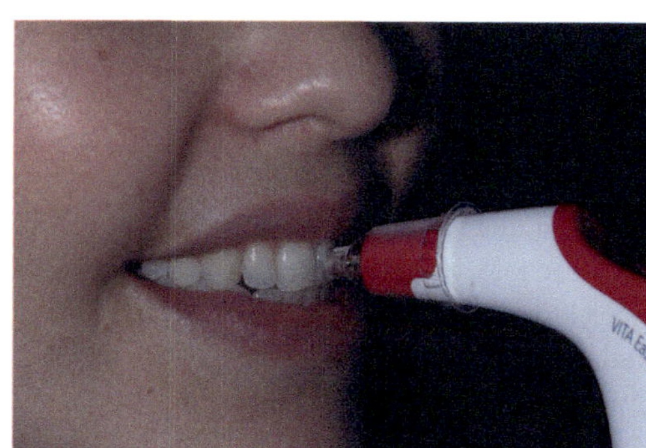

Fig. 4.6 Clinical use of the VITA Easyshade V spectrophotometer

Colorimeters measure tristimulus values and filter light in red, green, and blue areas of the visible spectrum. Although they have shown good measurement repeatability, they are subject to systematic errors due to the edge-loss effect related to sample surface, while spectrophotometers precisely measure color from reflectance or transmittance data [19, 40]. Colorimeters do not register spectral reflectance and can be less accurate than spectrophotometers (aging of the filters can additionally affect accuracy) [28, 41].

When analyzing the pros and cons of instrumental and visual methods, one can mention that instrumental methods such as spectrophotometers and colorimeters can help standardize color shade matching. On the other hand, they require specific and expensive technology, not always available to the clinician. On the other hand, a shade guide used to perform a visual shade matching method is always available in dental offices. However, this method is more subjective and operator dependent. A recent study showed that the spectrophotometer can assist with visual shade matching but cannot replace it [42]. Ideally, the combination of an equipment and visual shade matching should be used, and the help of a digital camera can promote successful results on shade matching [9, 27].

4.3.4 Digital Photography

Digital photographs can capture a detailed image of the tooth, be easily stored and transmitted to a technician, providing good quality information regarding color across the tooth surface, shape, and characteristic features. As will be further explored in Chap. 5, digital cameras have been increasingly used in dental offices to document the pre-operative situation, final results, and long-term outcomes [9, 27, 43]. A digital instrument capable of taking photographs, being it either a digital camera or a smartphone, is now available in all dental offices; thus, it is a technology that can be widely used.

Problematically, digital photographs of the natural dentition typically show significant color alterations of teeth and soft tissue when certain parameters are wrongly manipulated or when diffusers that filter the illuminant are used [27], for instance, changes in lighting conditions can result in changes in perceived color, and an incorrect digital camera exposure and automatic white balance can be reflected into an erroneously added cyan to the image to neutralize the high proportion of red tones from the gingiva while adding a tinge of blue to offset the yellow tones from the teeth [44]. For example, in soft tissues, a correct white balance can distinguish healthy from inflamed tissues. For hard tissues, correct color rendition reveals features such as enamel translucency, caries, erosion and abrasion, and cervical dentin exposure [45].

Flash photography also present differences within different types of flashes, even when used together with the same digital camera [27]. It was demonstrated that the combination of a digital camera with cross-polarization is the most standardized colored type of photography, although when performing the white balance of photographs using a gray reference card with known color values, a wireless close-up Speedlight flash showed to promote as standardized colored photography as with the use of a filter. The same was not observed for ring flashes, which tends to darken the images if they are not white balanced [27]. A recent study demonstrated that the problem caused by different diffusers in digital cameras could be compensated by using a gray reference card with known color coordinates to white balance the photographs [27], and although it did improve standardization of a digital camera when using a ring flash, it did not improve photographs made with a smartphone.

Smartphones are commonly available instruments, which have self-contained central processing unit (CPU) computing capability, enriched functionalities, software applications, wireless connectivity, and can present high-resolution photographic technology [46]. A recent publication showed that with novel appropriate light-correction filters, shade selection with the smartphone and the digital camera were comparable, showing to be reliable for shade selection, with ΔE values below the acceptable threshold [9].

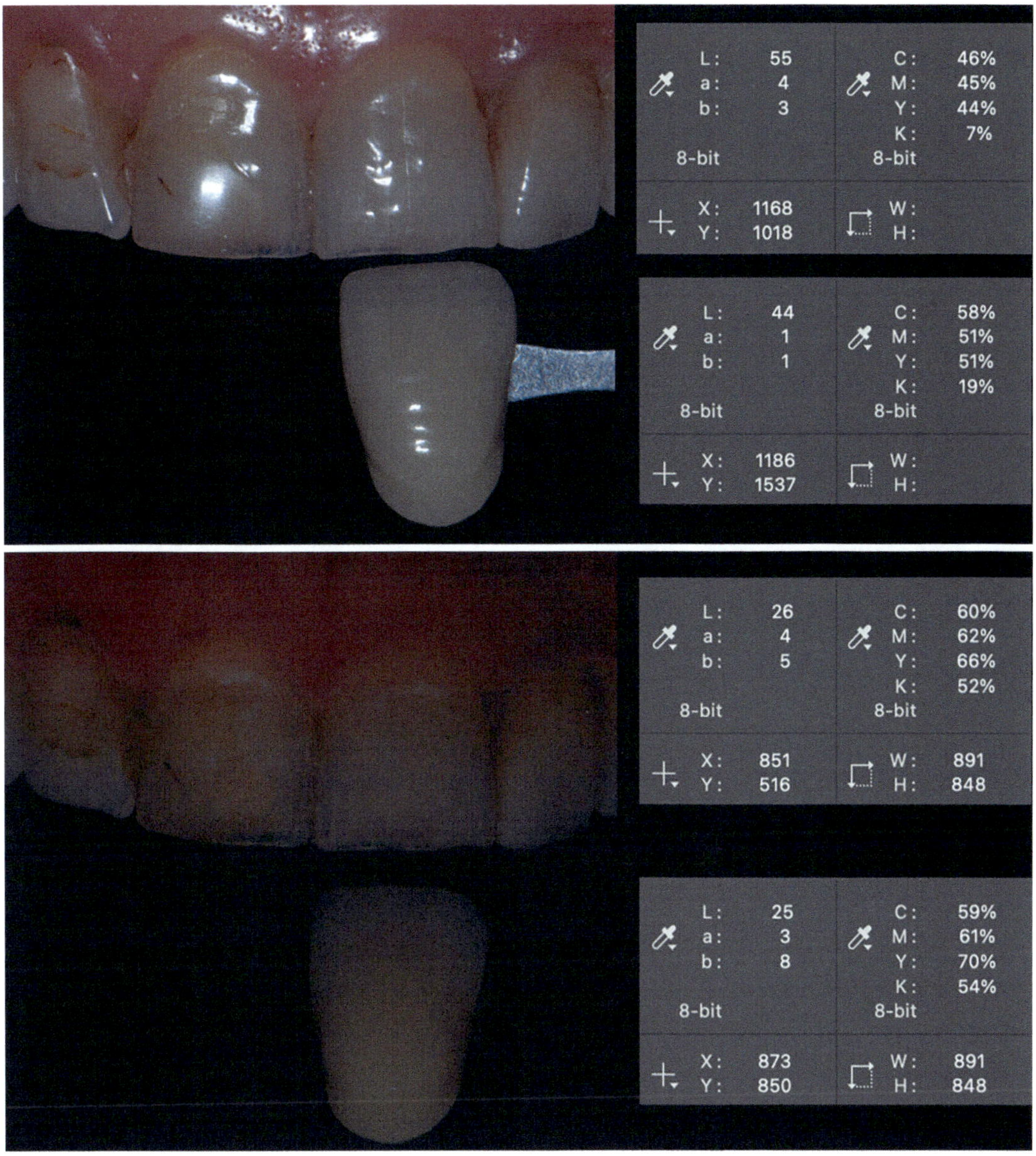

Fig. 4.7 Use of the Adobe Photoshop software to describe color values without (upper image) and with (lower image) the use of a cross-polarizing filter. Observe that total CIE-Lab values greatly vary between the photos

Thus, when using digital photograph, it is important to white balance the photographs using a gray reference card with known color values, which can be done using a software (for example, Lightroom v6.0, Adobe Photoshop CC; Adobe Systems Inc), or combining the use of a conventional photograph with one using a cross-polarizing or a light-correction filter. This technique is further explored in Chap. 5. The use of this software can also describe the color values in different color spaces, such as the CIE-Lab color space (Fig. 4.7). Moreover, both digital camera and smartphone photographs can be easily manipulated to observe tooth color and textures (Fig. 4.8).

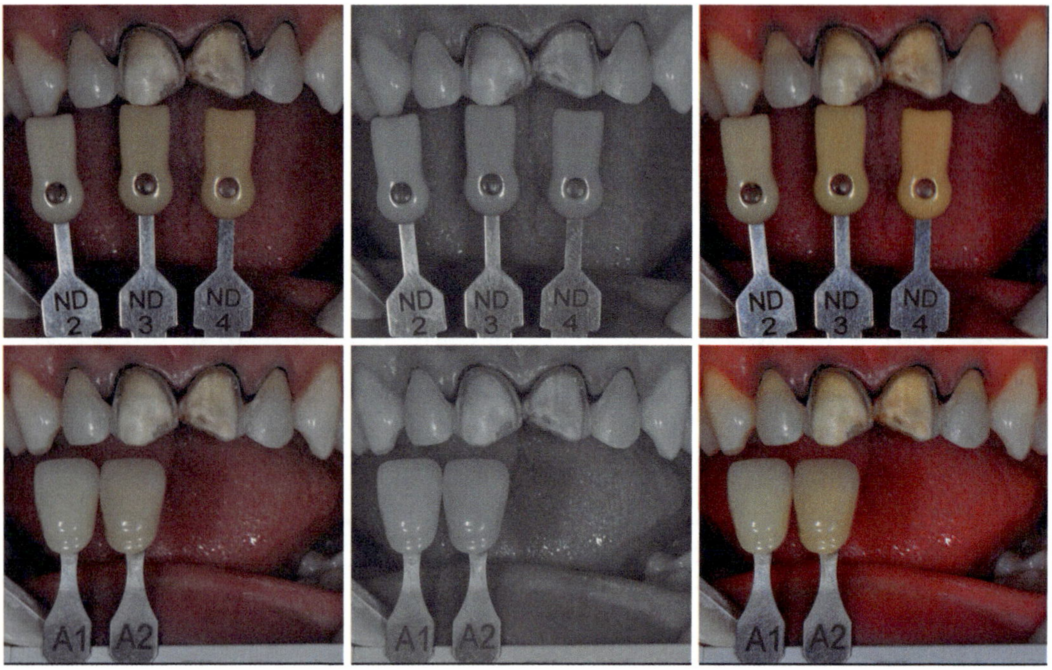

Fig. 4.8 Digital photographs used for digital shade selection taken with a digital camera, after manipulation with a digital software in different contrasts. First row: photograph with teeth and substrate shade guides; second row, black and white; third row, saturated. Manipulating the photographs helps on observing different structures of the teeth, as well as the luminosity

4.4 Experimental Designs to Evaluate Color

4.4.1 Clinical Trials

When dealing with clinical trials, it is extremely important to only start the research after obtaining an approved consent from the participants and approval of an Ethical Committee.

When performing clinical trials where shade matching needs to be obtained, observers need to be tested and calibrated for color matching competence, irrespective of their experience and demonstrate superior color discrimination competence according to ISO/TR 28642:2016 [25]. It is important that operators perform blind evaluations, and it is paramount to standardize illumination and background appropriately, as will be mentioned below. Also, in the visual analysis of color differences, a ranking can be used to compare, for instance, the color between a tooth and restoration, which can be graded. For example: from 0 to 4, using the scale based on a previous study where level "0" means excellent match; 1, very good match; 2, not so good match (border zone mismatch); 3, obvious mismatch; and 4, huge (pronounced) mismatch [20, 21].

An important aspect when dealing with natural teeth is dehydration. Tooth dehydration makes teeth appear whiter due to increasing enamel opacity. The interprism spaces become filled with air instead of water, so light can no longer scatter from crystal to crystal. Therefore, loss of translucency due to dehydration causes more reflection, which masks the underlying color of dentin, making the tooth appear lighter. Also, it has a negative impact on shade selection, which can affect the final esthetic outcome [47]. Shade selection procedures should be carried out within the first minute of the procedure and before teeth dehydrate [47]. Although it is frequent to observe dentists waiting for the tooth to rehydrate for shade taking, a recent study observed that teeth do not rehydrate within 15 min after rehydration; thus, it is important that shade selection is carried out in controlled circumstances before the tooth dehydrates [47].

4.4.2 In Vitro Studies

The same as mentioned previously in the clinical studies, when dealing with in vitro studies that use human tissues, first of all, it is extremely important to only start the research after obtaining the approval of an Ethical Committee. An extremely important topic is to always standardize illumination and background when evaluating the in vitro samples, which will be discussed below.

When compared to clinical studies, in vitro studies have the advantage of simulating specific procedures in an aged situation. For instance, the color stability of different materials can be assessed without actually needing to wait years until the material deteriorates. Instead, thermocycling procedures can be used to assess the color stability after simulated aging. Such procedures can be performed conventionally, in water, or even in different types of beverages. While if the same study was performed in mouth, it would take a long period of time to deteriorate, when aged in vitro, such results can be obtained within days [48, 49]. Another method of accelerated aging is using ultraviolet light. Studies have shown a yellowing effect after this type of aging due to a large positive change in b^* [33]. For all these types of studies, both visual and digital methods can be used, and color values, as well as color differences, can be obtained with the previously mentioned color difference (ΔE) formulas, as well as instrumental devices.

Different software can be used for the evaluation of colors in dentistry in vitro. Among all, the most commonly used is Adobe Photoshop, which can describe color values in different color scales, such as the CIE-Lab scale. Another interesting and easy access software used in recent research projects is the Classic Color Meter, which describes color values in the CIE-Lab scale [9, 27].

4.4.3 Illumination

For both in vitro and in vivo research, color evaluation and shade matching should be done using standardized color temperature illumination. The specific color temperatures range within 5000 (D50)–7500 K (D75) and are sought because of their universal nature and a broad spectrum of wavelength [48]. Nevertheless, such conditions are rare to be found since daylight is always changing and can range from 1000 to 20,000 K, making it difficult to rely only on natural daylight to provide the "ideal" color temperature during shade selection for a restoration [14].

For simulation of the ideal illumination for research, different apparatuses can be used. For instance, viewing booths and color boxes can be used for standardizing lightning and analyzing shade colors [14], handheld lights and provide significant improvements on shade matching [14], cross-polarizing filters (Fig. 4.9) used together with digital cameras can also provide more color-standardized photographs [27], a light-correcting device used with a smartphone also showed to be reliable for shade selection, with DE values below the acceptable threshold [9].

4.5 Background

The background is defined as the surface upon which samples are placed along with the environment [25]. The neutral light gray background has been recommended in the literature as the most appropriate for background and/or surrounding area in dentistry [27]. Today, white balance reference cards with known color coordinates are available in the market and can be used together with dental photography backgrounds. They have been recommended for improving standardization and accuracy in recording, communicating, and manipulating color images in dental digital photography [9, 27]. Besides a gray card itself, photographic contrastors are also available for both research and clinical basis; they can be found in different colors, such as black, simulating the dark background of the mouth, and gray, for a neutral background and white balance promotion (Fig. 4.10) [49].

In dental practice, the background is represented most often by the darkness of the oral cavity; nevertheless, there are situations when the shade selection is performed against other artifacts [17]. A recent study selected different backgrounds/surrounding area to simulate the different clinical situations, such as gray (considered as neutral and most frequently recommended), white (simulating color of opposite teeth), black (simulating color selection against a black contraster), red (imitating the lips and oral mucosa), and blue (simulating the rubber dam). Color matching results recorded against the blue background were statistically worse than to other backgrounds, while white and black generated the best results [17].

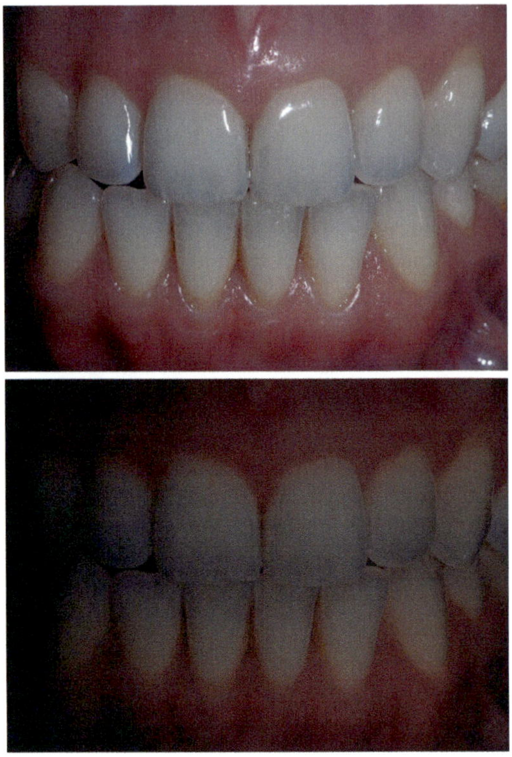

Fig. 4.9 Upper photograph taken without a cross-polarizing a filter, lower photograph taken with a cross-polarizing filter. Observe the absence of specular reflections in the photograph with filter, which allows a more straightforward and precise observation of natural teeth internal structures

4.5.1 Sample Size and Statistics Analyses

Statistical analyses are paramount in both clinical trials and in vitro studies. There is a necessity to organize and record the information obtained in the form of numbers from each sample. The value that is taken by the variable is called data, which can be classified into continuous data (Quantitative) or categorical data (Qualitative) (Figs. 4.11 and 4.12) [50].

When talking about color evaluation for research purposes, we will mainly work with continuous variables, where color values using mathematical formulas described in this chapter are made on a scale. This kind of data will be presented in terms of mean ± standard deviation. The recommended way to represent the final out-

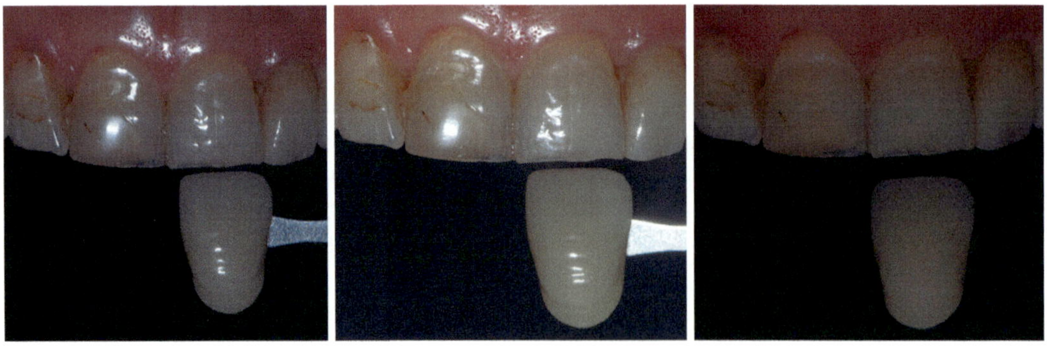

Fig. 4.10 Tooth color selection performed against a black background, gray background, and with a cross-polarizing filter

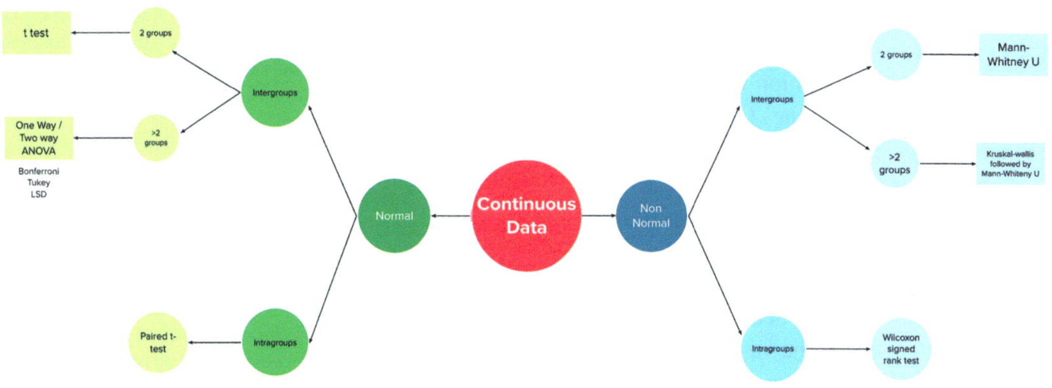

Fig. 4.11 Some of the most used statistical tests for continuous data

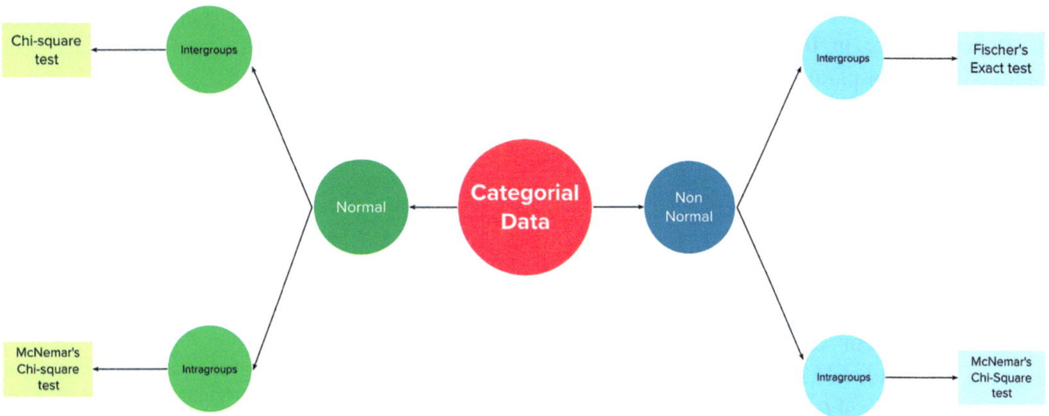

Fig. 4.12 Some of the most used statistical tests for categorical data

comes of any given test is in the form of tables and graphs.

The distribution of the data does not have a relation with the quality of the obtained data itself [50]. Distribution is just the pattern of values obtained [51]. Both empirical and theoretical distributions can be found; the most common theoretical distribution is the normal distribution, which is just a name and does not imply normality. For a normally distributed dataset, the majority of the sample's values or observations (95%) will be in the center of the distribution. Recommended tests to evaluate the normality of the data are the Kolmogorov–Smirnov test and the Shapiro–Wilk test. Usually, the Shapiro–Wilk test will be the appropriate method for small sample sizes (<50 samples), while the Kolmogorov–Smirnov test will be used for larger sample sizes (≥50 samples). In both cases, the null hypothesis is that the data falls within a normally distributed population when $p > 0.05$. The null hypothesis is accepted; therefore, the data are called normally distributed [52].

It is key in statistics that all the assumptions of the desired test to be performed are fulfilled. Normality is assumed in correlation, regression, *t*-test, and analysis of variance. Whenever there is a Normally distributed dataset, a parametric test can be used; if this condition is not met, then the use of a non-parametric test is required. Non-parametric tests include Wilcoxon signed-rank test, the Mann–Whitney *U* test, and the Kruskal–Wallis test.

Among the most commonly used tests, there is the Bonferroni test, which is intended to use for a small number of comparisons (<5), however, when dealing with larger than five comparisons, the preferred test is the Tukey test [50]. When the sample sizes and population variances are different between groups, the Games–Howell and Dunnett's tests give accurate results [50].

Other recommended tests that authors have used in studies involving clinical measurements are repeated measurements tests, where time-invariant unobservable differences between individuals can be controlled. This allows the researcher to estimate the variations within individuals. Here is where linear models come into play to fit the data, assuming that the distribution is Normal. Other linear models involve linear mixed models which are used when there is nonindependence in the dataset. On the other side, when a non-parametric test is required, the option would be to use generalized estimating equations (GEE) which includes subject-specific random effects.

This method also assumes that the values are correlated so that cases are not independent; for example, when performing multiple color measurements over time, compare different treatments or different color measuring methods. Figures 4.11 and 4.12 summarizes some of the most used statistical tests.

For statistical analysis, the preferred software to use due to its interface is SPSS (IBM). Hence, it is always advised to have a prior consultation with a statistician to match the data, analysis, and conclusions.

References

1. Paravina RD, O'Neill PN, Swift EJ Jr, Nathanson D, Goodacre CJ. Teaching of color in predoctoral and postdoctoral dental education in 2009. J Dent. 2010;38:e34–40.
2. Bergen SF, Paravina RD. Color education and training in dentistry: a first-hand perspective. J Esthet Restor Dent. 2017;29(2):E3–5.
3. Ristic I, Stankovic S, Paravina RD. Influence of color education and training on shade matching skills. J Esthet Restor Dent. 2016;28(5):287–94.
4. Paravina RD, Pérez MM, Ghinea R. Acceptability and perceptibility thresholds in dentistry: a comprehensive review of clinical and research applications. J Esthet Restor Dent. 2019;31(2):103–12.
5. Sproull RC. Color matching in dentistry. Part I. The three-dimensional nature of color. J Prosthet Dent. 1973;29(4):416–24.
6. Felippe LA, Monteiro S Jr, De Andrada CAC, Di Cerqueira AD, Ritter AV. Clinical strategies for success in proximoincisal composite restorations. Part I: understanding color and composite selection. J Esthet Restor Dent. 2004;16(6):336–47.
7. Villarroel M, Fahl N, De Sousa AM, de Oliveira OB. Direct esthetic restorations based on translucency and opacity of composite resins. J Esthet Restor Dent. 2011;23(2):73–87.
8. Sproull RC. Color matching in dentistry. Part III. Color control. J Prosthet Dent. 1974;31(2):146–54.
9. Jorquera GJ, Atria PJ, Galán M, Feureisen J, Imbarak M, Kernitsky J, et al. A comparison of ceramic crown color difference between different shade selection methods: visual, digital camera, and smartphone. J Prosthet Dent. 2021. https://doi.org/10.1016/j.prosdent.2020.07.029
10. Igiel C, Lehmann KM, Ghinea R, Weyhrauch M, Hangx Y, Scheller H, et al. Reliability of visual and instrumental color matching. J Esthet Restor Dent. 2017;29(5):303–8.
11. Paravina RD. Performance assessment of dental shade guides. J Dent. 2009;37:e15–20.
12. Paravina RD, Powers JM, Fay RM. Dental color standards: shade tab arrangement. J Esthet Restor Dent. 2001;13(4):254–63.
13. Sampaio CS, Gurrea J, Gurrea M, Bruguera A, Atria PJ, Janal M, et al. Dental shade guide variability for hues B, C, and D using cross-polarized photography. Int J Periodontic Restor Dent. 2018;38:113–8.
14. Clary JA, Ontiveros JC, Cron SG, Paravina RD. Influence of light source, polarization, education, and training on shade matching quality. J Prosthet Dent. 2016;116(1):91–7.
15. Pecho OE, Ghinea R, Perez MM, Della BA. Influence of gender on visual shade matching in dentistry. J Esthet Restor Dent. 2017;29(2):E15–23.
16. Haddad HJ, Jakstat HA, Arnetzl G, Borbely J, Vichi A, Dumfahrt H, et al. Does gender and experience influence shade matching quality? J Dent. 2009;37:e40–e4.
17. Dudea D, Gasparik C, Botos A, Alb F, Irimie A, Paravina RD. Influence of background/surrounding area on accuracy of visual color matching. Clin Oral Investig. 2016;20(6):1167–73.
18. Di Murro B, Gallusi G, Nardi R, Libonati A, Angotti V, Campanella V. The relationship of tooth shade and skin tone and its influence on the smile attractiveness. J Esthet Restor Dent. 2020;32(1):57–63.
19. Perez MM, Ghinea R, Herrera LJ, Carrillo F, Ionescu AM, Paravina RD. Color difference thresholds for computer-simulated human Gingiva. J Esthet Restor Dent. 2018;30(2):E24–30.
20. de Abreu JLB, Sampaio CS, Benalcázar Jalkh EB, Hirata R. Analysis of the color matching of universal resin composites in anterior restorations. J Esthet Restor Dent. 2020;33(2):269–76.
21. Pereira Sanchez N, Powers JM, Paravina RD. Instrumental and visual evaluation of the color adjustment potential of resin composites. J Esthet Restor Dent. 2019;31(5):465–70.

22. Wagner S, Rioseco M, Ortuño D, Cortés MF, Costa C. Effectiveness of a protocol for teaching dental tooth color in students with color vision impairment. J Esthet Restor Dent. 2020;32(6):601–6.
23. Bratner S, Hannak W, Boening K, Klinke T. Color determination with no-match-templates using two different tooth color scales—an in vitro evaluation. J Esthet Restor Dent. 2020;32(6):593–600.
24. Paravina RD, Ghinea R, Herrera LJ, Bona AD, Igiel C, Linninger M, et al. Color difference thresholds in dentistry. J Esthet Restor Dent. 2015;27:S1–9.
25. ISO/TR 28642:2016. Dentistry—Guidance on colour measurement; 2016.
26. Takatsui F, de Andrade MF, Neisser MP, Barros LAB, de Loffredo LCM. CIE *L** *a** *b**: comparison of digital images obtained photographically by manual and automatic modes. Braz Oral Res. 2012;26(6):578–83.
27. Sampaio CS, Atria PJ, Hirata R, Jorquera G. Variability of color matching with different digital photography techniques and a gray reference card. J Prosthet Dent. 2019;121(2):333–9.
28. Chu SJ, Trushkowsky RD, Paravina RD. Dental color matching instruments and systems. Review of clinical and research aspects. J Dent. 2010;38:e2–e16.
29. Paravina RD, Swift EJ Jr. Color in dentistry: match me, match me not. J Esthet Restor Dent. 2009;21(2):133–9.
30. Ghinea R, Pérez MM, Herrera LJ, Rivas MJ, Yebra A, Paravina RD. Color difference thresholds in dental ceramics. J Dent. 2010;38:e57–64.
31. Paravina RD, Westland S, Kimura M, Powers JM, Imai FH. Color interaction of dental materials: blending effect of layered composites. Dent Mater. 2006;22(10):903–8.
32. Commission Internationale del É clairage. CIE Technical Report: Colorimetry. CIE Pub No. 15.3. Vienna ACCB.
33. De Oliveira DCRS, Ayres APA, Rocha MG, Giannini M, Puppin Rontani RM, Ferracane JL, et al. Effect of different in vitro aging methods on color stability of a dental resin-based composite using CIELAB and CIEDE 2000 color-difference formulas. J Esthet Restor Dent. 2015;27(5):322–30.
34. Paul SJ, Peter A, Rodoni L, Pietrobon N. Conventional visual vs spectrophotometric shade taking for porcelain-fused-to-metal crowns: a clinical comparison. J Prosthet Dent. 2004;92(6):577.
35. Khurana R, Tredwin C, Weisbloom M, Moles D. A clinical evaluation of the individual repeatability of three commercially available colour measuring devices. Br Dent J. 2007;203(12):675–80.
36. Kielbassa AM, Beheim-Schwarzbach NJ, Neumann K, Zantner C. In vitro comparison of visual and computer-aided pre-and post-tooth shade determination using various home bleaching procedures. J Prosthet Dent. 2009;101(2):92–100.
37. Lagouvardos PE, Fougia AG, Diamantopoulou SA, Polyzois GL. Repeatability and interdevice reliability of two portable color selection devices in matching and measuring tooth color. J Prosthet Dent. 2009;101(1):40–5.
38. Paul S, Peter A, Pietrobon N, Hämmerle C. Visual and spectrophotometric shade analysis of human teeth. J Dent Res. 2002;81(8):578–82.
39. https://www.vita-zahnfabrik.com.
40. Chu SJ, Paravina RD, Sailer I, Mieleszko AJ. Color in dentistry: a clinical guide to predictable esthetics. Hanover Park: Quintessence; 2017.
41. Kim-Pusateri S, Brewer JD, Davis EL, Wee AG. Reliability and accuracy of four dental shade-matching devices. J Prosthet Dent. 2009;101(3):193–9.
42. Pecho OE, Ghinea R, Alessandretti R, Pérez MM, Della BA. Visual and instrumental shade matching using CIELAB and CIEDE2000 color difference formulas. Dent Mater. 2016;32(1):82–92.
43. Hein S, Zangl M. The use of a standardized gray reference card in dental photography to correct the effects of five commonly used diffusers on the color of 40 extracted human teeth. Int J Esthet Dent. 2016;11(2):246–59.
44. Snow SR. Assessing and achieving accuracy in digital dental photography. J Calif Dent Assoc. 2009;37(3):185–91.
45. Casaglia A, De Dominicis P, Arcuri L, Gargari M, Ottria L. Dental photography today. Part 1: basic concepts. Oral Implantol. 2015;8(4):122.
46. Tam W-K, Lee H-J. Accurate shade image matching by using a smartphone camera. J Prosthodont Res. 2017;61(2):168–76.
47. Suliman S, Sulaiman TA, Olafsson VG, Delgado AJ, Donovan TE, Heymann HO. Effect of time on tooth dehydration and rehydration. J Esthet Restor Dent. 2019;31(2):118–23.
48. Curd FM, Jasinevicius TR, Graves A, Cox V, Sadan A. Comparison of the shade matching ability of dental students using two light sources. J Prosthet Dent. 2006;96(6):391–6.
49. https://smilelineusa.com.
50. Krithikadatta J, Valarmathi S. Research methodology in dentistry: part II—the relevance of statistics in research. J Conserv Dent JCD. 2012;15(3):206.
51. Altman DG, Bland JM. Statistics notes: the normal distribution. BMJ. 1995;310(6975):298.
52. Mishra P, Pandey CM, Singh U, Gupta A, Sahu C, Keshri A. Descriptive statistics and normality tests for statistical data. Ann Card Anaesth. 2019;22(1):67.

5 Dental Photography as a Key to Clinical Success

Lucas Fernando Tabata, Toni Arcuri, and Leandro Augusto Hilgert

Much of dental treatment success relies on efficient communication between professionals and patients, among members of the professional team, along with the laboratory prosthesis technician involved in the treatment. Dental photography allows us to capture details and share certain aspects of a clinical case, such as tooth shape, texture, color, and perceived translucency [1, 2]. Furthermore, it enriches the communication between work team and patient since they enable us to capture smile harmony, the exposure of the incisal edge with resting lips, gingival exposure, and oral corridor. Photographs have become an essential tool in dentistry, as they have improved the way we communicate and relate to people. Besides documenting cases and assisting in planning treatments, dental photography also offers the possibility of reviewing the treatment performed to enhance and evolve our skills. DSLR (digital single-lens reflex) cameras are currently the gold standard in dentistry for providing high-quality results, on top of the ease of sharing the images and videos obtained. However, with technological development, more straightforward digital cameras such as smartphones and compact cameras have become a viable entry level option for the world of dental photography. Understanding how a digital camera works and knowing the differences between the various cameras and accessories available is imperative. As is acquiring knowledge on their advantages and limitations, knowing how to adjust the settings of your equipment, and mastering the concepts and fundamentals of photography. Grasping these core aspects will help you obtain even better images.

5.1 Digital Cameras

There are currently several types of digital cameras available for use in dentistry from different manufacturers. They each bear its own characteristics, indications, and limitations, and can be classified into five distinct groups as presented in the image below (Fig. 5.1).

5.1.1 Smartphones

Smartphone cameras have evolved significantly in the recent years, as have devices and their processors in general. Instead of using lenses with optical zoom—which would compromise the thickness of phones—most manufacturers have incorporated multiple lenses. High-end smartphones have three lenses (ultra-wide, wide, and

L. F. Tabata (✉) · L. A. Hilgert
Department of Dentistry, School of Health Sciences, University of Brasilia, Brasilia, DF, Brazil
e-mail: leandrohilgert@unb.br

T. Arcuri
School of Dentistry, Uniceplac University, Brasilia, DF, Brazil

D. Oliveira (ed.), *Color Science and Shade Selection in Operative Dentistry*,
https://doi.org/10.1007/978-3-030-99173-9_5

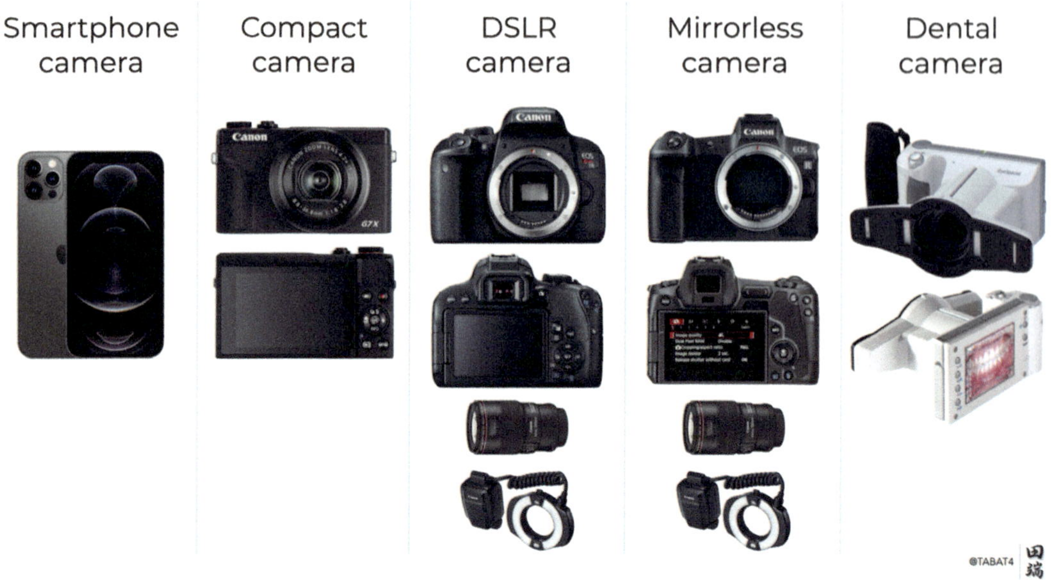

Fig. 5.1 Classification of digital cameras

telephoto lens) that can be easily selected according to each specific situation. However, even with the versatility of using multiple lenses, the image capture sensors in these devices are still small. They tend to obtain more pixelated images when greatly enlarged or in low light environments. Some devices feature a pro mode or manual mode, which allows for the adjustment of settings. When this function is not present, there are specific downloadable apps for this purpose. Even though they do not have a dedicated macro-lens, their portability and accessibility make them excellent entry option to start capturing dental photographs, despite their limitations.

Recommendation: if you opt to use a smartphone for dental photography, since they do not include a dedicated macro-lens, we suggest opting for a model with multiple lenses (Fig. 5.2). Remember to check that one of the lenses is a telephoto lens. If your smartphone does not offer a telephoto lens option, you can use the digital zoom of your device, mindful that this will lower the resolution of image. The use of telephoto lens or digital zoom causes less image distortion since wide and ultra-wide lenses tend to change the photographed object's proportion, known as the barrel distortion. Another critical point for capturing good quality dental photographs is the use of an external continuous light source, such as LED panels or an LED ring light. This allows brighter images to be obtained and avoids high noise in the image by the camera's ISO (sensitivity) compensation.

5.1.2 Compact Cameras

Developed to be portable and user-friendly, these were the first digital equipment accessible to the general public, that associated the digital technology of the time with affordability. Also known as point-and-shoot cameras, they had added features to facilitate usage. These properties included automatic mode, autofocus, retractable zoom lenses, built-in flash, and video recording, making them very popular since the beginning of the year 2000. Nowadays, some compact cameras even feature a manual mode for configuring camera settings and, along with smartphones, they are an excellent entry level choice for the world of dental photography.

Recommendations: if present, we recommend using the camera in manual mode, with the macro-function activated, employing the optical

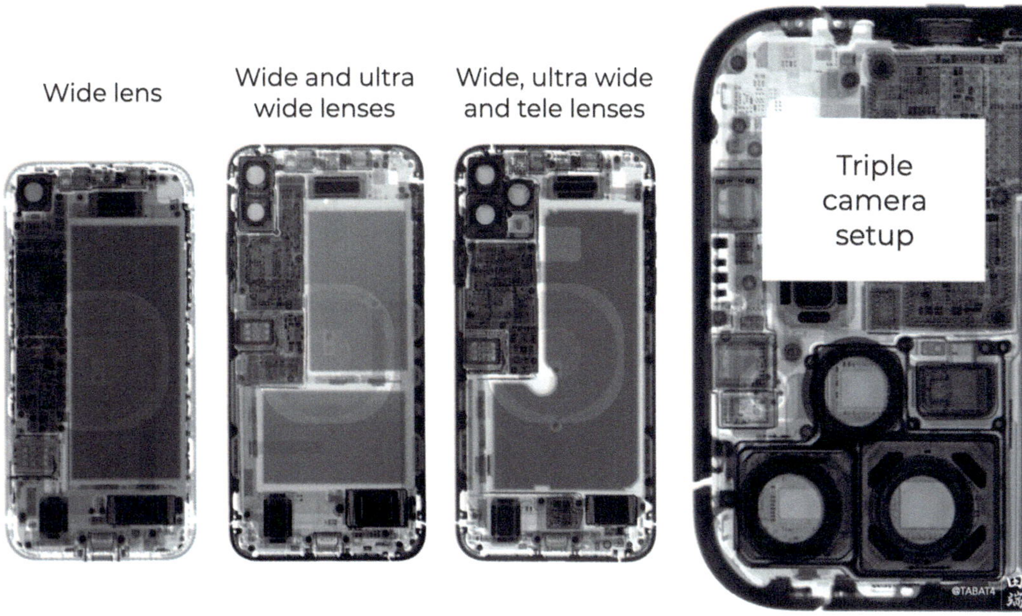

Fig. 5.2 X-ray of smartphones showing the digital camera components. (Adapted from https://www.creativeelectron.com/)

zoom lens to reduce image distortion. It is recommended to combine it with an LED illuminator or an external flash to synchronize with camera's shutter, whenever available.

5.1.3 DSLR (Single-Lens Digital Reflection)

DSLR cameras are characterized by using a pentaprism (reflex mirror) to visualize the object before the photographic record occurs. These are often considered professional or semi-professional cameras, which employ full-frame or APS-C type sensors to capture images with excellent resolution and high quality. Another key feature is the possibility of adjusting the equipment's settings to manual mode. This optimizes the capture of images and grants the operator total control over the photograph to be obtained. The use of an interchangeable lens (Fig. 5.3) and an external flash as an auxiliary source of illumination, makes this equipment the gold standard for dental photography, especially when the goal is to attain high-quality images. This feature grants users the ability to adapt to different situations. We recommend using a dedicated macro-lens from 100 to 105 mm and a circular or twin macro-flash.

5.1.4 Mirrorless Cameras

Considered an evolution of DSLRs and cameras, they present the same possibility of using interchangeable lenses and external flashes. The main difference is the absence of the pentaprism (reflex mirror) inside the camera body, which allows this equipment to be smaller and lighter than the DSLRs. Instead of the optical viewfinder, these cameras enable digital previewing of the image on a built-in rear LCD screen or an electronic viewfinder (EVF). A disadvantage of mirrorless cameras when compared to a typical DSLR is its shorter battery life, due to the power consumption of the viewfinder. However, an in-camera setting on some models can mitigate this issue. With more technology involved, they still have higher cost, which should become more accessible over time.

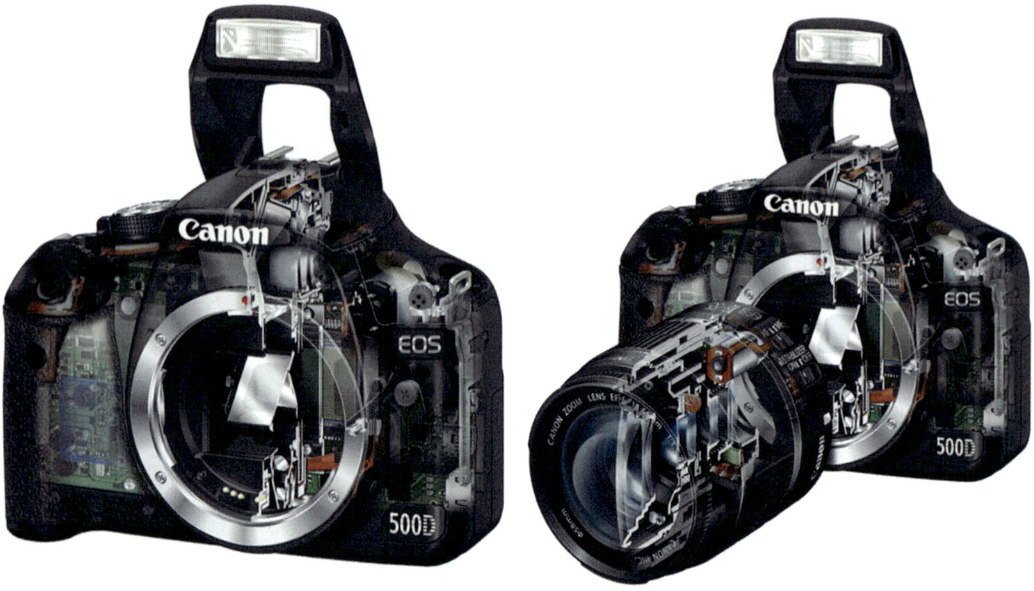

Fig. 5.3 Schematic illustration of a DSLR equipment. (https://www.dpreview.com/articles/6579860130/canoneos500d)

We recommend using a dedicated macro-lens from 100 to 105 mm and a circular or twin macro-flash.

5.1.5 Specific Cameras for Dentistry

There is also on the market a digital dental camera designed exclusively for dentistry (EyeSpecial C-IV, SHOFU, JAPAN), which incorporates the advantages of DSLR cameras with the simplicity of compact cameras. It features software with a user-friendly interface, touchscreen and the menu offers pre-configured modes. Among its advantages is the body. Its lightweight unibody construction in polymer is resistant to moisture and disinfection protocols, favoring biosafety within the office space. It features a dual twin flash integrated into the camera body, which is selected according to the pre-configured modes. There is also a 28–300 mm lens with the option of adding a close-up lens for macro-photography, and an adapter for cross-polarized photography for photos of color selection.

We advise using the pre-configured modes recommended by the manufacturer, since the equipment is specific for dentistry.

5.2 Knowing the Photographic Equipment and Accessories for Dental Photography

5.2.1 Sensor

Sensors are responsible for capturing the light reflected by an object, which will later be processed to acquire the desired photographed image. There are two main types of image sensors for digital cameras and camcorders: CMOS and CCD. Both are made of silicon and work in similar way. They depend on the photoelectric effect, the interaction between photons (particles of light) and the silicon, to move the electrons in the sensor to capture the image. All these sensors are charge-coupled devices and their basic functions are to capture images and transform them into electrons (electromagnetic signals) and bits and bytes by a microprocessor in an analog-digital process that generates the image. The main difference among equipment resides in the type and size of sensor used (Fig. 5.4). Professional DSLR cameras use full-frame sensors, while intermediate and entry level DSLRs use APS-C sensors (1.5–1.6x smaller than the full-frame sensor). Compact cameras use 1″

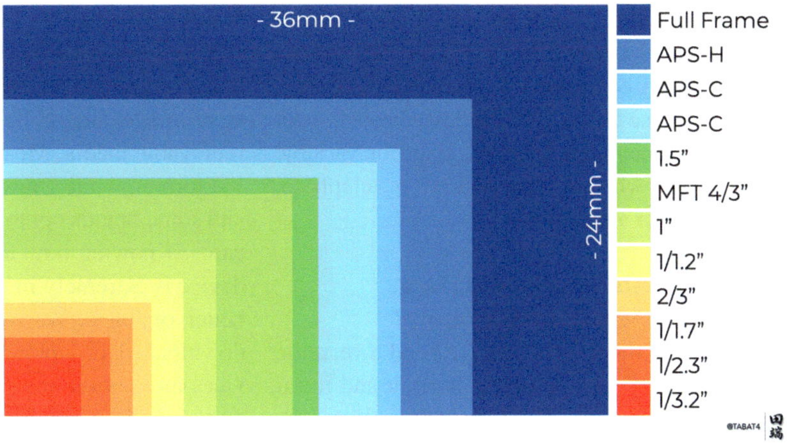

Fig. 5.4 Comparison of the size of the digital sensors used in photographic equipment. (Adapted from https://newatlas.com/camera-sensor-size-guide/26684/)

sensors, while smartphones use 1/3″ sensors, almost 50 times smaller than the full-frame sensor.

5.2.1.1 How Important Is the Size of the Sensor?

A digital camera's resolution is often limited by the image sensor that turns light into discrete signals. Depending on the sensor's physical structure, a color filter array may be used, which requires demosaicing to recreate a full-color image. The brighter the image at a given point on the sensor, the higher the value read for that pixel. The number of pixels in the sensor determines the camera's "pixel count." In a typical sensor, the pixel count is the product of the number of rows and the number of columns. For example, a 1000 by 1000 pixel sensor would have 1000,000 pixels or 1 megapixel. In practice, while smaller sensors tend to produce more pixelated and noisier images, larger sensors capture more defined images. These present superior color contrast and performance in a low light situation, lower noise at high ISOs, and lower crosstalk.

5.2.2 Camera Body

The framework is responsible for maintaining and protecting the sensor and processor, along with supplemental electronic equipment, that together allow the camera to function. The body's size may vary between equipment based on the amount and size of electronic components. Larger bodies provide space for larger sensors and enable better handling and grip. In DSLR or mirrorless cameras, it is possible to connect a single lens and flashes to the equipment's body. Not all compact cameras include these options, and it is not possible to exchange lenses. Only a few models offer the possibility to connect an external flash to the camera body. In smartphones, the camera body is integrated with the mobile itself, which, like compact cameras, offers little possibility of adapting direct lenses and synchronizing flashes as DLSRs and mirrorless do.

5.2.3 Lens

A lens is composed of several optical elements, which can be made of plastic or glass. Optical glass elements generally provide a clearer, higher-quality lens result. Each element has a specific function in focusing the light towards the sensor, either generally shaping the light to fit the sensor's size, correcting problems, or providing the final point of focus. An interesting feature of these lenses is the automatic focus. In this case, a motor's aid allows for the final optical element or collection of some elements to be moved closer or farther from the sensor. This enables different areas of an image to appear in focus and is one of the main aspects of a practical camera system. The lens can be considered the most important element of a camera. Aspects such as number, size, and configuration of optical elements, material quality, number of blades in the diaphragm, and electronic components, determine its characteristics. These characteristics have direct impact on clarity, maximum aperture, fixed or variable focal length, whether wide, macro, or telephoto, and manual or autofocus.

5.2.3.1 Which Lens Should I Use for Dental Photography?

In everyday clinical practice, we need a versatile lens that allows us to perform portrait and intraoral close-ups with minimal distortion (Fig. 5.5). For this purpose, dedicated macro-lenses for DSLR or mirrorless cameras have been the gold standard in dentistry. It is important for the focal length to be between 100 and 105 mm, depending on the manufacturer, to allow for a 1:1 magnification. For devices that do not offer the possibility of using interchangeable lenses, such as compact cameras and smartphones, we suggest using the camera's optical zoom, whenever possible, or the telephoto lens on a smartphone (Fig. 5.6). Otherwise, digital zoom can be used, with the understanding that this will decrease the resolution of the image.

5.2.4 Memory

Some smartphones and most digital cameras store image data on flash memory cards or other removable media. Most stand-alone cameras use SD format, while a few use CompactFlash cards, and some brands opt to use their specific memory cards. Knowing how files are stored inside your device is extremely important, as it allows you to better organize. We recommend that photos be downloaded or uploaded to cloud storage services more often on smartphones that rely solely on the device's internal memory. It is important to note that adopting a file organization protocol is crucial to keep track of your cases. Whenever necessary, consider using an external hard drive to backup your digital files.

5.2.4.1 Which File Format Should I Use?

The Joint Photography Experts Group (JPEG) standard is the most common file format for storing image data. Other file possibilities include Tagged Image File Format (TIFF) and several RAW image formats. Raw image is the unprocessed set of pixel data directly from the camera sensor, often saved in a proprietary format. Many

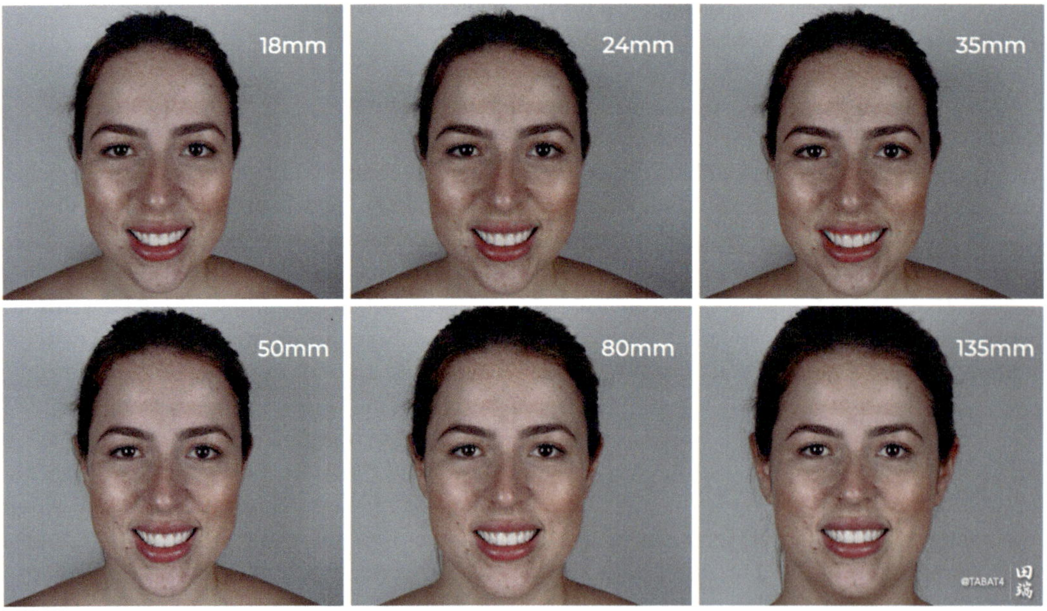

Fig. 5.5 Display of barrel distortion. Barrel distortion is usually present in most lenses, especially at wide angles. The distortion amount can vary, depending on the distance between camera and object, especially over short distances

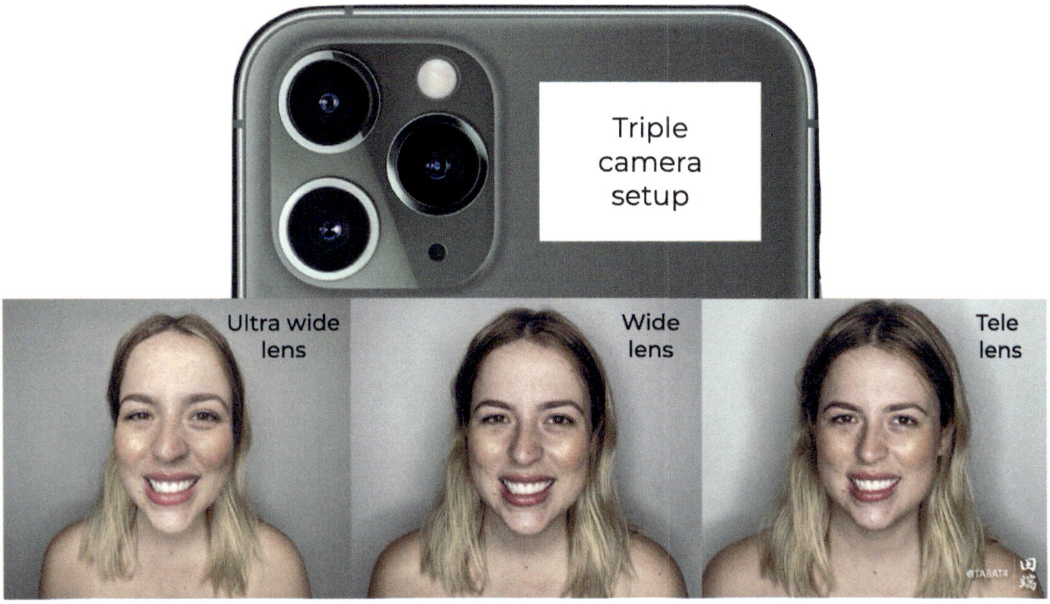

Fig. 5.6 Display of barrel distortion present in smartphones

cameras, especially high-end ones, support a RAW image format. At first, RAW files had to be processed in specialized image editing programs but, over time, many conventional editing programs, such as Google's Picasa, added support for RAW images. Rendering to standard images from RAW sensor data grants more flexibility when making major adjustments without losing image quality or retaking pictures. In general, it is relevant to consider that the RAW format will be necessary when you intend to enlarge a picture for printing, or even in cases where it is necessary to prove copyright. Another instance when this might be needed is to confirm the absence of image editing, as well as in cases of communication of shade selection with a laboratory technician. For this purpose, we recommend the use of a gray card associated with a cross-polarizing filter which will be later explained in this chapter. When sharing patient's image in clinical routine, JPEG format will suffice.

5.2.5 Lighting Equipment for Dental Photography

Light is the main ingredient for photography and are classified as natural or artificial. In this chapter, we will cover those of interest to dentistry, which are artificial lights. There are four common types of artificial light sources used in photography: incandescent, fluorescent, LED, and flash. For dentistry purposes, we will deal with the latter two (Fig. 5.7). In dental photography, we work with artificial light from lighting equipment classified as continuous light equipment or flash-type equipment. While both options illuminate and provide better results in filming and photographing, they present some technical differences, such as the "time" in which the light is available. Continuous light is an option that promotes continuous lighting over timer, while with flash, lighting occurs punctually. Other factors such as color temperature and light intensity

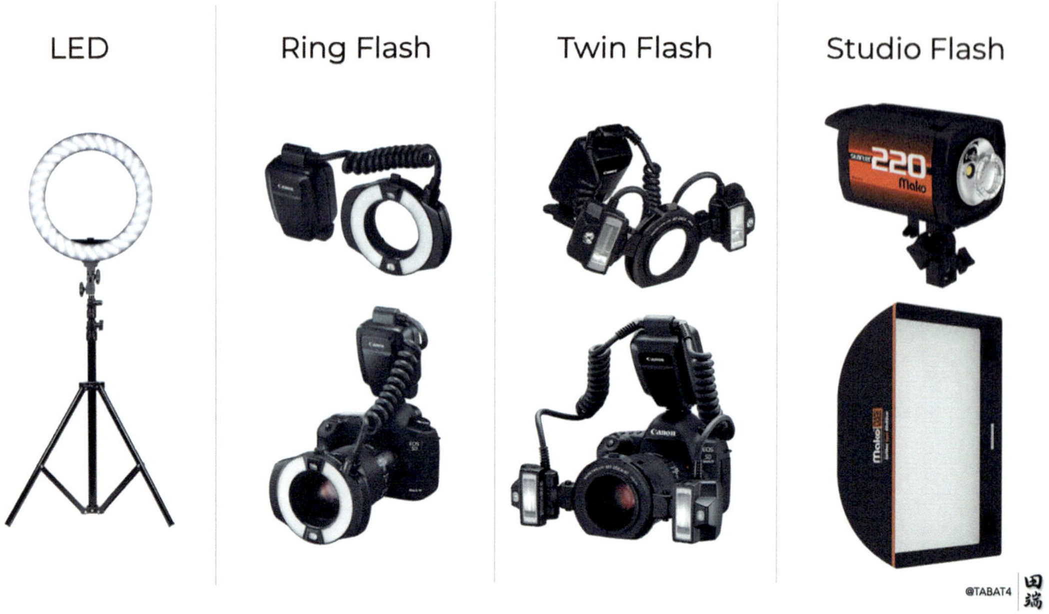

Fig. 5.7 Artificial lighting equipment available for use in dental photography

should also be considered when choosing between these options.

5.2.5.1 Continuous Light Equipment

LED means light-emitting diodes. The light source in such devices is generated by a series of light-emitting diodes present in each lamp. These illuminators are classified as continuous light equipment because the light remains on the entire time and does not flash like a strobe light. Most LED equipment offers brightness adjustment for the emitted light, as well as color temperature adjustment option, which ranges from 3300 (yellowish light) to 6600 K (white light), for example. Since LEDs are not as bright as the light emitted from a flash light, they are not recommended for taking photographs with DSLR or mirrorless cameras. However, it is possible if you use a high ISO setting (800+) or position them very close to your subject.

Despite that, LED illuminators are effective with smartphone cameras and compact cameras (Fig. 5.8) since the camera's shot cannot be synchronized with the flash device in this case. Another interesting possibility of using LED equipment is while filming. Whether with DSLR, mirrorless, compact, or smartphone cameras, a continuous light source is always needed.

5.2.5.2 Flash Equipment

Photographic flash, sometimes referred to as a strobe or simply a flash, is a device used in photography to allow pictures of dark areas to be taken by producing an extremely bright light. This illumination is not continuous and, in a small fraction of a second, it bursts outward in large amounts. Most photographic equipment includes built-in flash, but external flashes will be needed for dentistry purposes since they enhance the lighting system. A critical factor when using this light source is the need to synchronize the firing of the photographic flash with the digital camera's shutter opening, to enable light to be captured by the electronic image sensor. In DSLRs and mirrorless cameras, the mechanism is usually a programmable electronic timing circuit, which can, in some equipment, receive input from a mechanical shutter contact or work wirelessly.

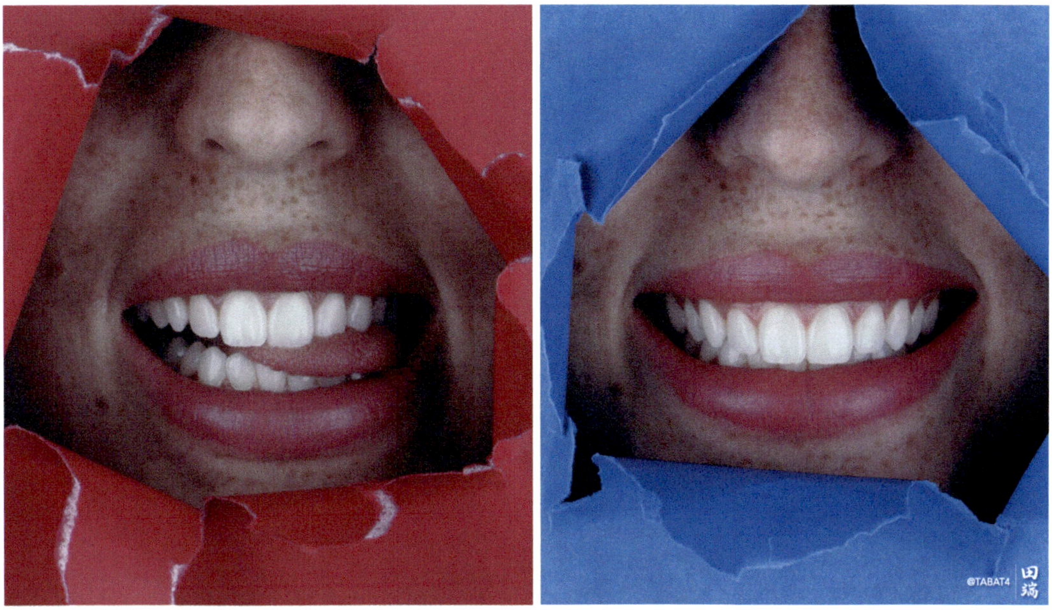

Fig. 5.8 Artistic photography was obtained using studio flash and a DSLR camera equipped with a 100 mm macro-lens

5.2.5.3 Macro-Flash for DSLRs and Mirrorless

For dental photographs, based on equipment configuration adjustments (which will be later discussed in this chapter), and due to the need to capture close-up photographs of subjects, built-in flashes are not recommended as they create shadows in the image. Instead, macro-flashes, like ring light and twin flashes, should be your first option for such situations. The advantage of these flashes is the ability to position the light source at the same plane as the lens, which provides better lighting for dental photos. An alternative to macro-flashes is the use of a pair of conventional external flashes, mounted on a bracket or on tripods, that are activated in remote mode to function as a twin flash or a studio flash. A critical factor when using these sources is the need to correctly set the light's intensity. This can be controlled automatically or in manual mode by the operator, providing greater control over the final result of the image.

5.2.5.4 Studio Flash

Another option that has become very attractive to clinicians is the use of studio flash equipment within the dental office. There are currently different models on the market, which can be mounted on tripods or attached to the dental office's ceiling. These models have greater power than macro-flashes and work plugged in, allowing for a faster firing cycle and less variety of light intensity since they do not depend on batteries. Studio flashes are generally combined with softboxes or umbrellas, which help diffuse the light from the flash, and provide softer shadows in the images, with a more artistic appeal (Fig. 5.8).

5.2.6 Light Modifying Accessories

The main objective of modifying the light of a photographic flash is to soften shadows. Since the photographic flash is a small, high-intensity light source, it usually produces harsh, unattractive shadows. Hard light directly affects the photographed object, by causing a well-marked and sharp shadow. Unlike with hard lights, the shadows generated by soft lights are absent of sharp edges, making it impossible to determine exactly where the shadow begins or ends (Fig. 5.9).

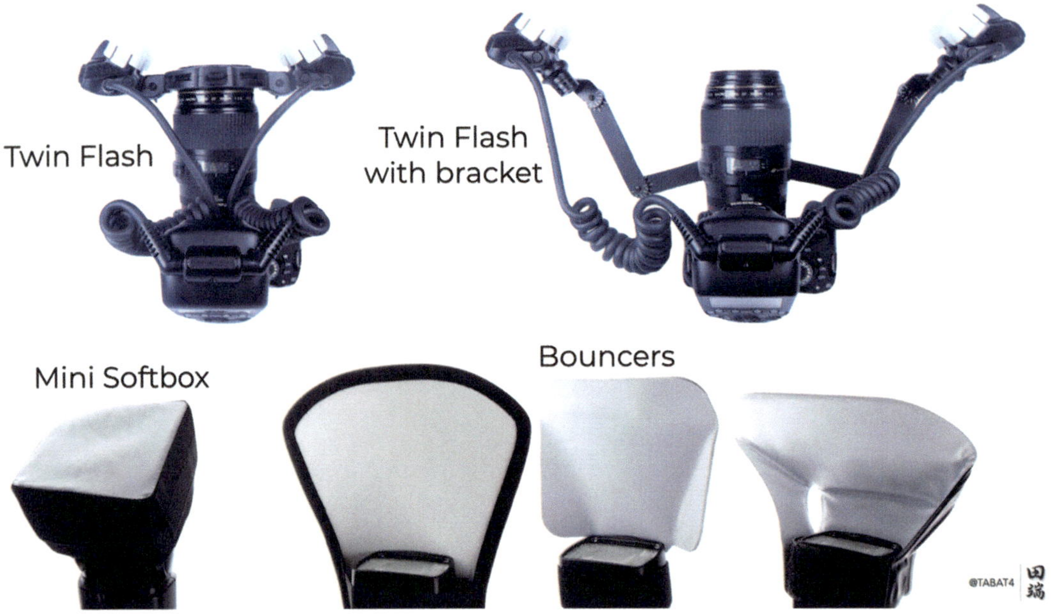

Fig. 5.9 Light modification accessories

5.2.6.1 Softboxes and Bouncers

There are two ways to "soften" the light from flashes: filtering or bouncing it, by using diffusers and reflectors, respectively, that work as light distribution devices. Flash diffusers soften shadows by refracting the light through a translucent material. When the light is refracted through a translucent material, this material becomes the new and the largest light source, as in the softboxes used in studio flashes. A simple and cheap solution is to attach a sheet of white paper over the twin flash with tape. In the case of reflectors, the light from the flash is directed to the reflectors' surface, which then reflects the light on its surface, and provides softer shadows. In practice, it is possible to soften shadows by using a light modifier that amplifies the light as a larger light source. This strategy produces a more gradual transition between deep shadow and full illumination. The most common misconception is that spreading the light over a wider area will soften the shadows. This is not the case. You must enlarge the light source to soften the shadows.

5.2.6.2 Brackets Mount

Another way to modify the light is to change the position of the light-emitting source or flash. For this, there are devices called brackets available, with option for fixed or articulated arms. These allow the twin flashes to be adjusted in different positions to increase distance or approximation of the light source concerning the subject and the camera lens. By modifying the flashes' positioning, indirect or oblique light are obtained enabling better visualization of the tooth's buccal surface texture. Since it provides more detailed information for laboratory procedures, this feature becomes very interesting when communicating with the laboratory technician. This bracket system can be used with conventional external flashes, along with remote mode and macro-twin flashes.

5.2.7 Accessories for Dental Photography

To perform good dental photographs, especially intraoral photographs, it is necessary to keep the lips, cheeks, and tongue out of the image The market has a variety of accessory models available that can be chosen from according to the photographic registration needs. Here we will address some possibilities and their practical applications (Fig. 5.10).

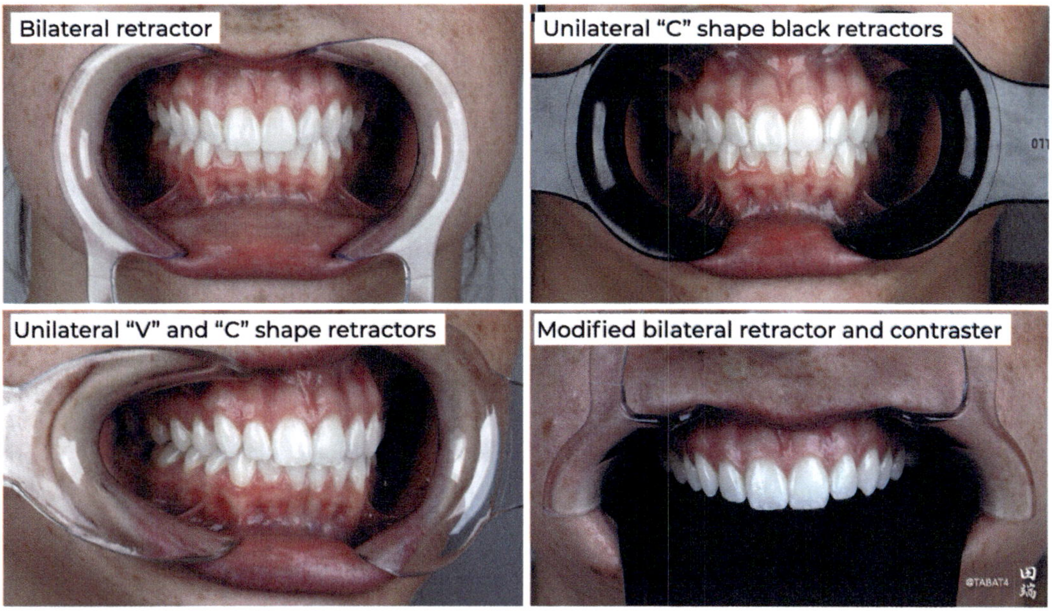

Fig. 5.10 For front photos, we recommend the use of a bilateral retractor, also known as self-retracting or unilateral retractors. For side shots, we suggest the use of an associated "V" shaped retractor (for the side to be photographed) and "C" shaped retractor (for the contralateral side). For occlusal photos, we recommend using a modified bilateral retractor with a mirror or an anterior photo with a black background

5.2.7.1 Mouth Retractors

Mouth retractors keep lips and cheeks out of the image. There are several mouth retractors available, which can be unilateral or bilateral, with C or V shape, transparent or colored. If necessary, we can modify retractors, mainly to optimize use when employing mirrors and black backgrounds.

5.2.7.2 Mirrors

A wide variety of mirrors are available for many intraoral situations, differing in size, shape, and the presence or not of a handle. These are essential for occlusal photos and can be associated with modified bilateral retractors for better results. Mirrors with handles help to ensure no fingers appear in the image. To prevent the mirror from fogging up due to the patient's breathing, we recommended the use air spray or preheating the mirror prior to performing the photoshoot.

5.2.7.3 Black Background

Black backgrounds or contrasters are used to isolate the anterior teeth, especially the upper teeth. When positioned behind the anterior teeth, the light from the flash is absorbed instead of reflected, enabling nuances of the tooth enamel to be observed, especially of the incisal edges and in the transition areas. This is very effective in communicating with the laboratory technician.

5.3 Fundamentals of Dental Photography: The Exposure Square

Dental photography is available to everyone. However, some basic principles about the dynamics of the equipment and the light's behavior are necessary and will be addressed in this section. After all, the etymology of the word photography does say it all: the art of drawing with light. From the Greek "phosgraphein"—"phos" or photo, which means "light," and "graphein," which means "to mark," "to draw" or "to register." The term "exposure" appears as a synonym for "making a photograph," and, from a technical point of view, it represents the amount of light that can reach the image recording medium [3].

5.3.1 Exposure

In photographs, exposure is responsible for capturing the amount of light that can reach the sensor of a camera. That is, it defines how light or dark photos will be. For instance, if the result of the image captured is very bright, it is because the image was overexposed, indicating "too much light." If it is too dark, it was underexposed, indicative of "low light."

Depending on the effect you are looking for, this may or may not be a good strategy. If the sensor receives a significant amount of light, the photo will be overexposed, with large white areas and the lack of details. In contrast, if the image sensor does not receive enough light, the photo will be underexposed, with black areas, yet also devoid of details. The ideal strategy to avoid missing details is to find balance.

In classic photography literature, three basic settings allow you to deal with the exposure of your photos: Shutter Speed, Aperture, and Image Sensor Sensitivity. These three configurations form what we call the Exposure Triangle. In Dental Photography, because we are dealing with the registration of a dark cavity that is not efficiently lit by ambient light, the use of flash is necessary and mandatory. Hence, when the Exposure Triangle of classical photography literature gains an additional pillar in Dentistry, it turns into an Exposure Square: the flash configuration (Fig. 5.11). All basic settings are interdependent, and each has a remarkable creative impact on the image.

5.3.1.1 Shutter Speed

Shutter Speed or exposure time translates into the time that the machine's shutter (the part that isolates the light sensor) remains open, letting the photographic film or the digital sensor absorb light and form an image. The longer the exposure time, the greater the absorption of light by the sensor, therefore the more exposed the image will be. Exposure time is usually given in $1/x$ format, where X represents a fraction of time in seconds. This component of the exposure triangle varies between 1/8000 of a second (very short time, higher speed) and several seconds (very long time, lower speed). Specifically, we can distinguish the short times (less than 1/60) from the long times (more than 1/60).

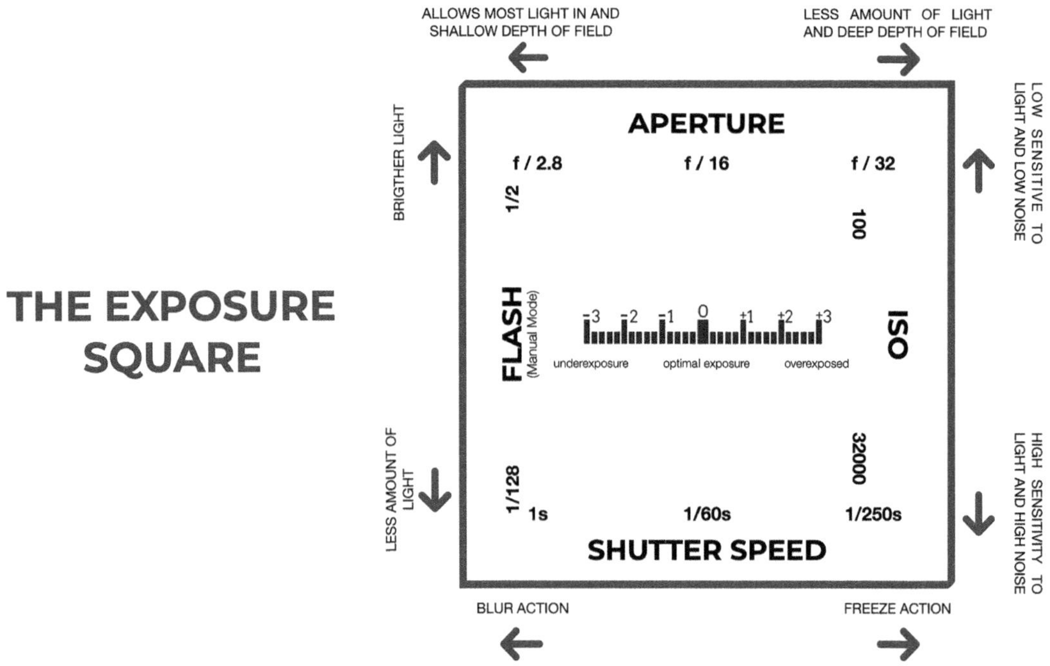

Fig. 5.11 The exposure square

Although very popular in the photographic field, the term speed is not correct. The shutter, as we have seen, works with exposure times, in general fractions of seconds, which does not relate to the speed of operation or exposure [4].

5.3.1.2 Impact of Shutter Speed on Image Blur

Shutter speed controls the effects of movement on your photos. This can occur deliberately, from the camera's movement by the photographer while recording an image, or from movements from your subject within your composition. Although fast shutter speeds freeze the action, slow shutters can register the action as a blur.

In Fig. 5.12, we can see three photos of the same pinwheel, taken of the object in motion, though with different exposure times. In conclusion, just remember, short exposure time causes a freezing effect of the motion of the subject to be photographed, while long exposure time causes motion blur or background.

5.3.1.3 Aperture

The camera lens contains a diaphragm, a type of membrane formed by a set of metal sheets, which can be closed more, or less, to allow greater or fewer light to pass through (Fig. 5.13). The wider the aperture, the more the image will be exposed.

Aperture is expressed by a number. The smaller the number, the greater the aperture. It is an inversely proportional relationship. For all lenses, the smallest aperture number (or f-stop)—1.4, 2, 2.8, or 4, depending on the lens—represents the largest aperture. The minimum aperture is often 22 at minimum focal lengths and can reach 38 or more.

5.3.1.4 Impact of Diaphragm Opening on Depth of Field

We call Depth of Field (DoF—Depth of Field) the area of the image that will be sharp, while the rest will be blurred. This Depth of Field depends on several factors:

1. *The opening of the diaphragm*: the more open the diaphragm, the smaller the depth of field.
2. *The long focal length*: long focal lengths (telephoto) tend to decrease the depth of field.
3. *The focus distance*: the closer the subject is, the smaller the depth of field.

For portraits, for example, a reduced depth of field is preferred so that the subject is sharp, but the background completely blurred. To do this, you need a lens with a large aperture (ex: f/1.8). We can also use zoom to take close-ups of the object so that it looks closer. It is a photographic

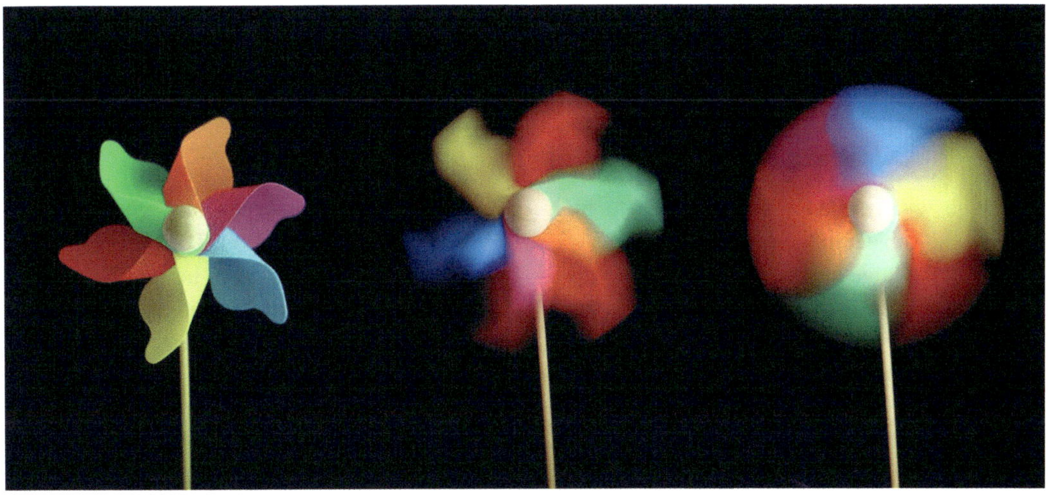

Fig. 5.12 Impact of the Shutter Speed on motion blur. (Adapted from https://digitalwarehouseblog.wordpress.com/2016/01/26/when-the-lights-go-down-low-light/)

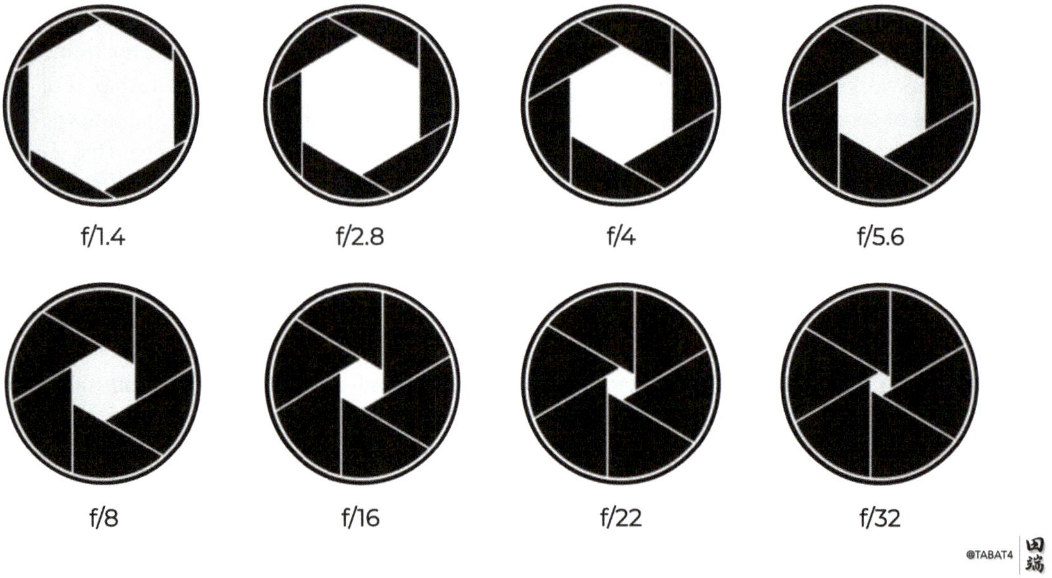

Fig. 5.13 Diaphragm and set of blades

Fig. 5.14 Reduced depth of field, showing in focus every tooth until the canine

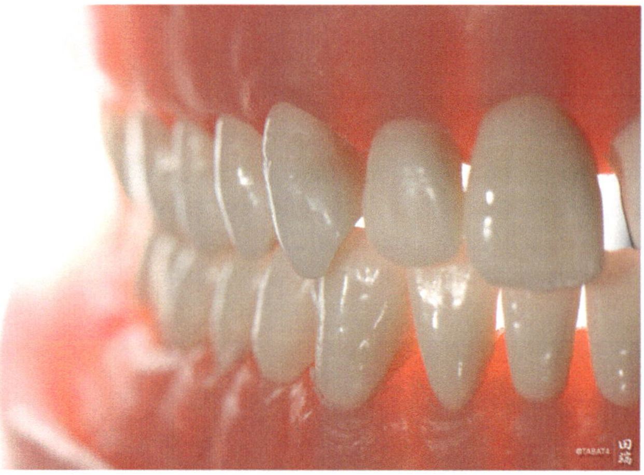

technique widely used when it comes to highlighting the subject in the foreground.

In short, a large aperture (small number) produces a reduced depth of field (small area of sharpness). A small aperture (large number) leads to a greater depth of field (area of deep sharpness). See Fig. 5.14.

5.3.1.5 Sensitivity (ISO)

The sensitivity of the image sensor (expressed in ISO—International Organization for Standardization) is the standard that describes the absolute sensitivity of the digital sensor to light, and it varies between 50 and 128,000. The higher the ISO, the lesser amount of light is needed to obtain a correct exposure since the sensitivity of the digital sensor to capture light will be grater.

The sensitivity of today's cameras reaches 128,000 ISO, and noise is almost invisible up to 3200 ISO. Noise can be defined as a kind of interference in the image that manifests itself in the form of pixels of very different colors from reality, usually in dark scenes [5] (Fig. 5.15).

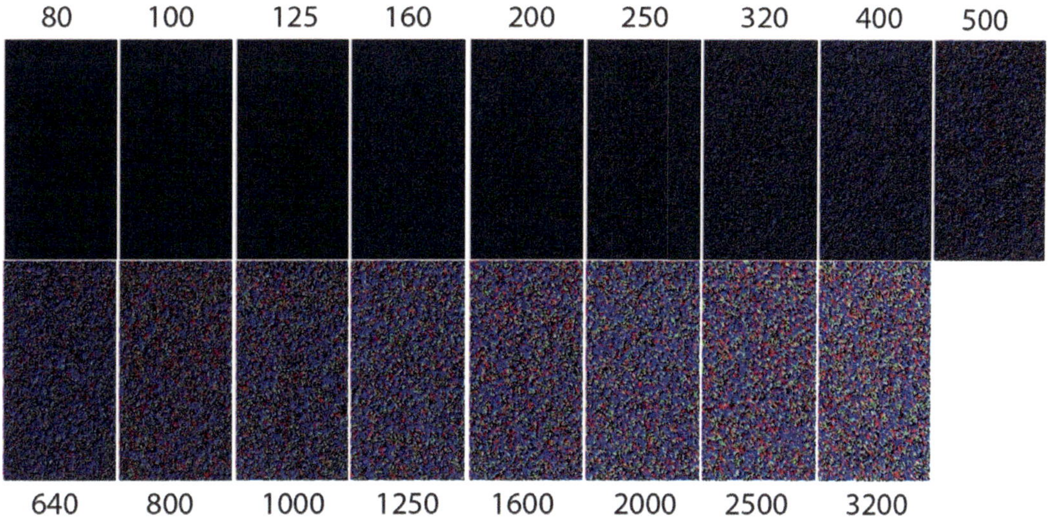

Fig. 5.15 ISO and noise production in the image

However, it is best to keep the ISO as low as possible: 100 ISO for sunny days, 200 ISO for cloudy days, and up to 400 ISO indoors. Nevertheless, if the scene demands it, do not hesitate to raise the ISO.

5.3.1.6 Impact of Sensitivity on Image Noise

As previously mentioned, increasing the ISO sensitivity can make photos lighter, however, it decreases the sharpness because it produces undesirable noise in the images due to the greater sensitivity to capture light.

It is recommended to maintain minimum sensitivity in Dental Photography. The ideal is to work with the ISO as low as possible, preferably in a range of 100–200, aiming to obtain images with the lowest possible level of noise and greater clarity. Any dark or shady area in the oral cavity can have its lighting issue resolved by using an integrated flash system specifically for this purpose.

5.3.2 Master the Exposure of Your Equipment

As we have seen, the correct adjustment of your equipment can favor obtaining better images. These settings adjustments may vary from equipment to equipment, depending on the type, model, and manufacturer. Below you will find a summary of general equipment configurations, though it is crucial that you carry out some tests with your equipment and adjust it according to your needs (Table 5.1 and Fig. 5.16).

5.4 Dental Photography with Gray Card

Gray cards are designed to help you adjust your exposure and white balance settings consistently, providing a reference point. This reference point will define a white balance or color balance point for a given image and all images subsequently captured. The reference point will ask your camera to compensate for any illuminating color in the space you plan to shoot, adjusting the white balance and the color profile (Fig. 5.17). With a gray card, it becomes possible to correct the values of color differences of dental elements to visually imperceptible values. This achieves one of the major advances in the standardization of photography for color registration. To measure your reference point, place the gray card in the area or scene where you intend to capture, with the gray side facing the camera. For most accu-

Table 5.1 Compilation of your equipment configuration recommendations

DSLR and Mirrorless	Compact Cameras	Smartphone Cameras
CAMERA MANUAL MODE • **F22** for better depth of field • **1/125** to avoid blur image • **ISO 100** for low noise • **WB** flash or use grey card for color correction FLASH MANUAL MODE • **1/2** to **1/4** MACRO LENS **100** or **105**mm • Autofocus or manual	• Use an external **LED light source** or flash equipment is possible to synchronise the shot. • Use optical **zoom** to decrease barrel distortion. • Select **macro** function. • **Adjust setup** on manual mode if possible.	• Use an external **LED light source.** • **Enable HDR** on your smartphone. • Use smartphone's **tele lens** or **digital zoom** to decrease barrel distortion. • Adjust setup manually on pro mode or using an app, or **adjust exposure** on your mobile screen. • To avoid shaky photos, use **timer** function.

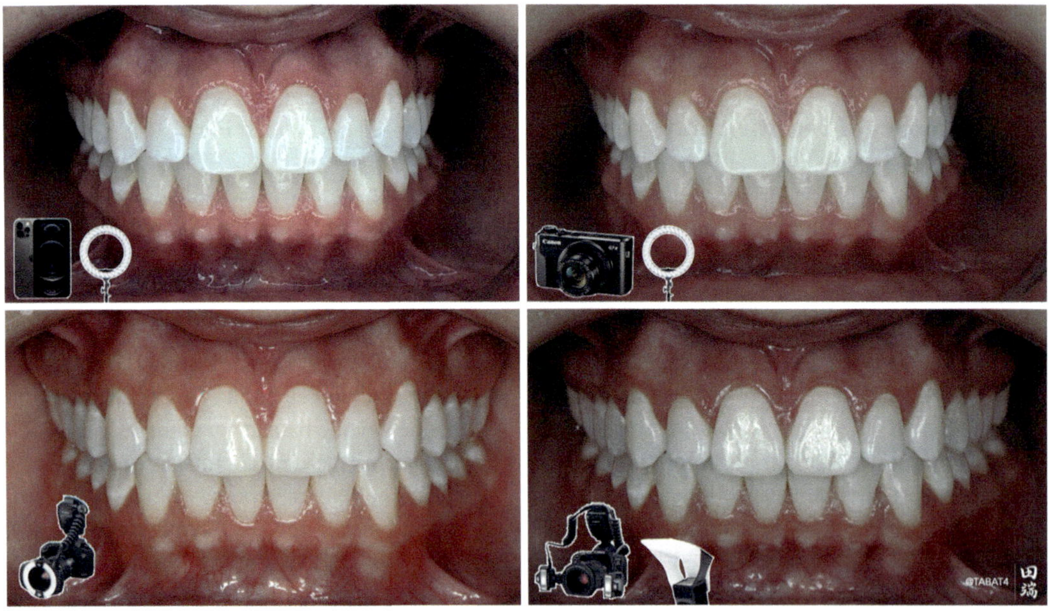

Fig. 5.16 Image results from smartphone plus LED (top left). Compact camera plus LED (top right). DSLR camera with a macro-lens and ring flash (bottom left). DSLR camera with a macro-lens and twin flash (bottom right)

rate results, place the card close to the patient's mouth so that it reflects the light from the flash. Then, adjust the white balance settings on the camera to ensure optimal exposure and focus. Shoot normally, remembering that you must repeat a new photo with the gray card whenever you change the lighting settings.

Another possibility is the post-processing procedure of white balance correction in software like Photoshop or Lightroom. To do so, merely

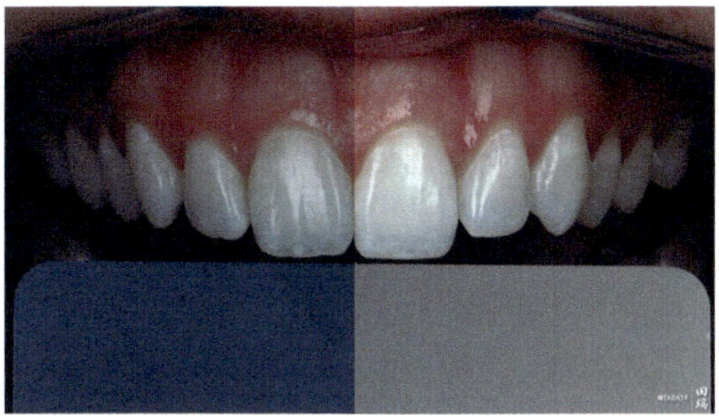

Fig. 5.17 The photograph was taken with a gray card (left side) and WB adjustment made in photoshop (right side)

open the test image that contains your gray card in Photoshop and create a Level Adjustment Layer. You will find three droppers stacked next to the Levels histogram. Select the middle dropper and click on the gray card. Photoshop will automatically adjust the color levels of the image for you. If you need to apply these settings to other images taken in the same lighting conditions, click on the drop-down menu in the upper right-hand corner of the Levels column and select "save preset levels." Name and save the preset, then open your other files for editing. For each image, find "load level preset" in the Levels column drop-down menu and select the saved preset file to apply it. To do this in Lightroom, simply select the White Balance dropper tool from the Developing Module Basic menu and click on the gray card. Then, highlight all the images you want to color and click on the "synchronize" button in the screen's lower right-hand corner. Check the "White balance" and click "synchronize."

5.5 Cross-Polarization in Dental Photography

For years, there were uncertainties regarding the ability of photographic captures to effectively register color shades of dental elements. These concerns related to the possibility of lighting affecting color, and to the potential of variations happening between the various sources of illumination. This was greatly attributed to possible variations and discrepancies occurring because of different photographic processes and the brand of the equipment. Some of the probable variances include intensities, degrees of angulation, distance, the use of modifiers, as well as the configuration of the camera and the differences between operators (dental surgeons, dental technicians, and dental assistants).

The human eye does not have the ability to distinguish between randomly oriented light and polarized light, and polarized flat light can only be seen through an effect of intensity or color. For example, by the reduced brightness when wearing polarized sunglasses. In fact, humans cannot differentiate real high contrast images seen in a polarized light microscope from identical images of the same specimen captured digitally (or on film) and then projected onto a screen with light that is not polarized.

The basic concept of polarized light is illustrated in Fig. 5.18 for a non-polarized light beam incident on two linear polarizers. Electric field vectors are represented in the incident light beam as sine waves that vibrate in all directions (360°; although only six waves, spaced at 60° intervals, are represented in Fig. 5.18). In reality, the electric field vectors of incident light are vibrating perpendicular to the direction of propagation, with an equal distribution in all planes before encountering the first polarizer [6].

The polarizers illustrated in Fig. 5.18 are filters containing long-chain polymer molecules oriented in a single direction. Only incident light vibrating in the same plane as the oriented polymer molecules are absorbed, while light that vibrates perpendicularly to the polymer plane passes through the polarizer. The polarization direction of the first polarizer is oriented vertically towards the incident beam so that only waves with vertical electric field vectors will pass through the first polarizer. The second polarizer, subsequently, blocks the wave that passes through the first polarizer because this polarizer is oriented horizontally concerning the electric field vector in the light wave. The concept of using two polarizers oriented at right angles to each other is commonly called Cross-Polarization and can be used with transmitted light (Transmitted Cross-Polarization—TCP) and reflected light

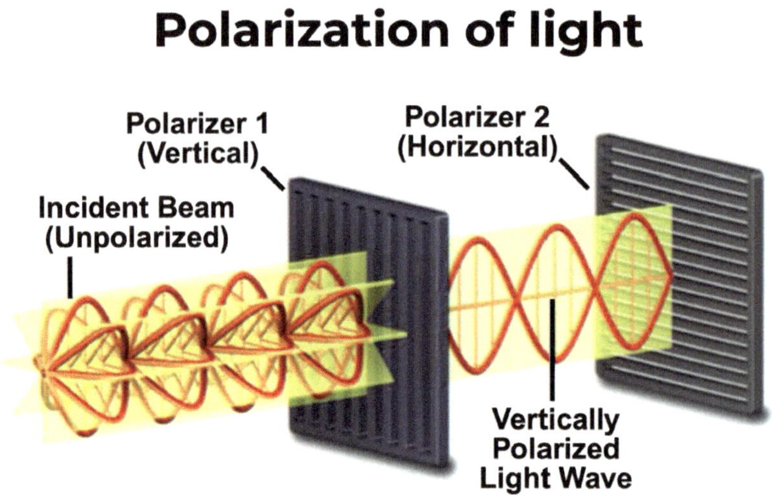

Fig. 5.18 Polarized light concept. (Source: https://www.microscopyu.com [7])

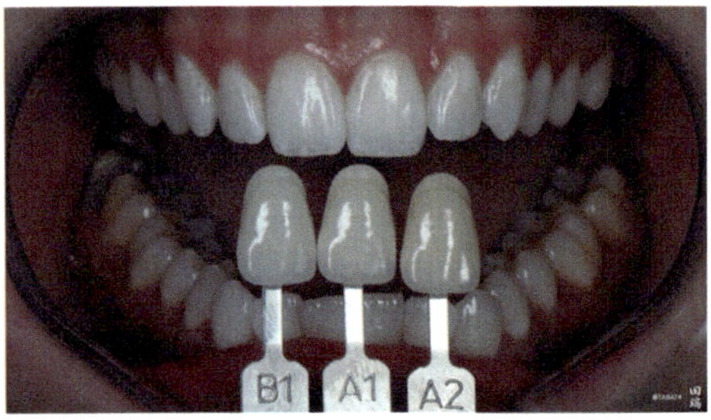

Fig. 5.19 Photo with color scale for communication with the laboratory. Note that the reflection of the flash interferes with the correct color analysis

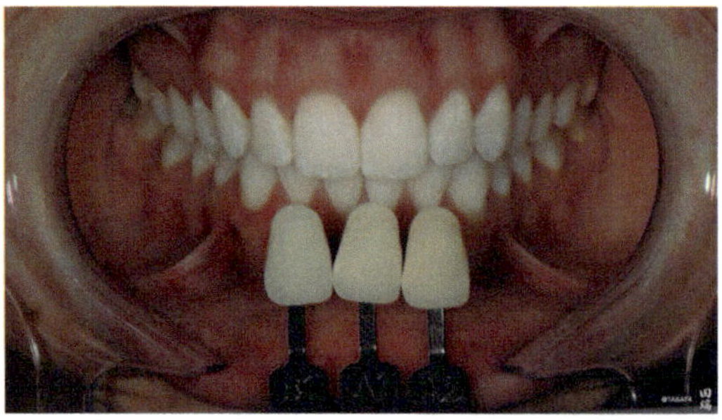

Fig. 5.20 Photo with the color scale using the reflected cross-polarization. By removing the flash light reflection, a better color evaluation of the patient's smile is possible

(Reflected Cross-Polarization—RCP). In photographs using the Transmitted Cross-Polarization, the light passes through the object to be studied and reaches the objective. In photographs using Reflected Cross-Polarization, the light falls on the object's surface to be studied and is then reflected towards the lens (Figs. 5.19 and 5.20).

5.6 Communication with the Laboratory

Color selection in dentistry is considered a subjective process, dependent on three factors: light source, object (tooth), and observer (dentist/patient/laboratory technician) [8]. Some studies [9–13] have been developed to try to standardize these factors using reflected polarized lighting and an absolute gray reference card, also called a white balance card.

The use of cross-polarized filters for dental photography allows the elimination of unwanted stray light and specular reflection from the dental structure from the buccal surface. These filters are incorporated into the flash and are located perpendicular to another polarizing filter located simultaneously on the front of the lens. This results in a high contrast image or a supersaturated image, allowing detailed chromatic mapping of the dental element (Figs. 5.21 and 5.22).

As demonstrated, the use of polarizing filters associated with digital photography is a simple and direct method used to better understand the color of the natural anterior dentition, improving communication with laboratory technicians, which makes the rehabilitation much more predictable (Fig. 5.23).

Sampaio et al. [10], compared the performance of different digital equipment and accessories for color selection. Among them were a smartphone, a DSLR camera with circular flash, a DSLR camera with twin flash, a DSLR camera with twin flash and light modifiers, and a DSLR camera with twin flash with polar eyes system, associated with the use of a gray card. They concluded that the use of gray cards favored results, optimizing the usage of digital equipment for color selection. The employment of reflected cross-polarization with the polar eyes system showed the best results and, according to this study, the smartphone was the least accurate.

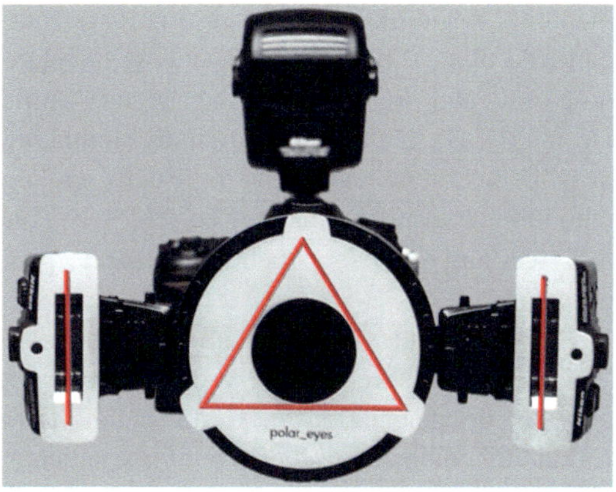

Fig. 5.21 Polar-eyes® cross-polarization filters. (Adapted from https://www.youtube.com/watch?v=uZwNKHnQyPw)

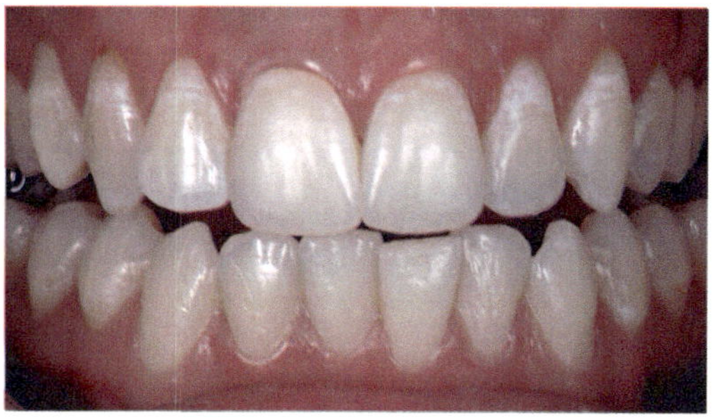

Fig. 5.23 Result achieved, harmonizing the element with a darkened substrate to the rest of the dental elements

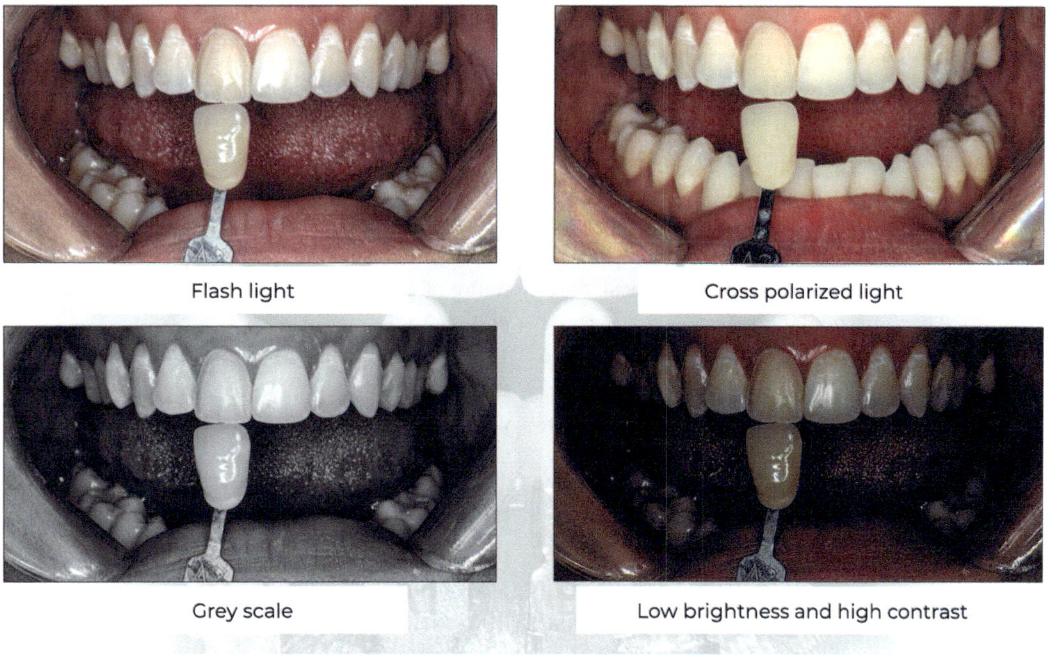

Fig. 5.22 The color taking of the substrate of the dental element, with the aid of reflected polarized light, for esthetic rehabilitation

As we mentioned at the beginning of this chapter, smartphones and compact cameras are still a long away from offering the same photographic quality achieved with DSLRs and mirrorless equipment. Nevertheless, these devices work for the entry level path in the world of dental photography and can be used until a better equipment can be acquired. Although they present some limitations (regarding sensor size and absence of a dedicated macro-lens), good results may be achieved with proper lighting and configuration setup. And indeed, a simpler picture of a clinical case performed with straightforward devices are better than no photo at all.

5.7 Photography in the Daily Practice of Dentistry

In the last decades, the evolution of digital cameras and accessories, its user-friendliness, larger accessibility, and lower costs, have exponentially increased the role of images in the dental practice quotidian.

Nowadays, it is possible to affirm that there is always a feasible way, regardless of budget, of recording dental treatment steps. Either by using an always present smartphone or a high-end camera with plenty of accessories, capturing relevant visual information opens a myriad of uses for the images. Quality will certainly vary according to the used equipment and the photographer's training and experience. Adjusting the needed equipment for one's routine is an exercise that, if well performed, will result in finding the best cost-benefit for each particular case.

The first reason to include photography in the dental practice routine to record patients' baseline and post-treatment images with the intent of documentation. It is also important for legal protection and for long-term follow-ups. As commonly said, an image is worth a thousand words. Nowadays with the availability of electronic files for patients, digital images can be easily attached and stored to records, enriching the documentation of treatment stages, and enhancing the level of recorded details.

In our experience, patients enjoy and value seeing on a screen (or even on the camera's LCD) what is being performed during treatment. A clinical picture can be a valuable instrument to increase patients' understanding of why certain procedures are needed, for educating patients on required behavioral changes, and for treatment planning. A well-known concept that uses standardized clinical pictures (and videos) for planning a dental treatment is the Digital Smile Design (DSD). It also allows digitally simulating possible treatment results and to visually explain (show) to the patient what may be achieved. This tool certainly aids esthetic treatment plan acceptance.

Post-treatment pictures, with or without an "artistic touch," are also very useful. And not only for documentation, or to allow long-term follow-ups comparisons, but to reinforce patients' perception of the dentists' work quality, which increases patients' fidelity.

Before and after photographs may also be used for marketing purposes. Be sure to always respect local regulations in terms of patients' privacy and all mandatory legal authorizations.

Well performed dental pictures greatly enhance the communication between dental professionals when discussing treatment plans and are valuable assets for educational and scientific purposes. Presenting clinical cases with images rich with relevant information, together with a solid scientific content, is the cornerstone of many of the best lectures at the main dental congresses of the world.

For those involved in prosthodontics, enabling the dental technician to see, in detail, the clinical case for which an indirect restoration will be produced is truly a must. Tooth color, shape, texture, and the singularities of each patient's tooth can be easily shared. Digital photography and, in present days, the commonly digital flux of restorative dentistry have surely increased the quality of exchanged information and reduced distances in the dentist/dental technician relationship. The use of standardized reference shade tabs, gray cards, calibrated monitors, and a good understanding of some of the dental photography concepts presented in this chapter on both the clinical and the laboratory ends of the process strengthen the level of communication [11].

On the topic of color, standardized digital photography—particularly those using concepts of exposure adjustment with a gray card and reflected cross-polarization—can be used not only to shade selection in prosthodontics [11, 12], but also for the quantification of color in clinical research [14].

5.8 Final Remarks

Dental photography is an inseparable part of modern Dentistry. In every dental specialty, predominantly those involved in esthetics, the use of images has increasingly gained relevance over the past years. Knowledge of the basics of the subject, such as required equipment, fundamentals of photography, and some practical training on achieving useful images, should be part of a contemporary dental curriculum.

References

1. Zyman P, Etienne JM. Recording and communicating shared with digital photography: concepts and considerations. Pract Proced Aesthet Dent. 2002;14(1):49–51.
2. Chu SJ, Tarnow DP. Digital shade analysis and verification: a case report and discussion. Pract Proced Aesthet Dent. 2001;13(2):129–36.
3. Santos JF. Luz, exposição, composição, equipamento. Farmalicão: Centro Atlântico; 2010.
4. Terry DA, Geller W. Esthetic and restorative dentistry: material selection and technique. Chicago: Quintessence; 2013.
5. Peterson B. Understanding exposure, fourth edition: how to shoot great photographs with any camera. New York: Amphoto; 2016.
6. Hallimond F, Taylor EW. An improved polarizing microscope. III. The slotted ocular and the slotted objective. Mineral Mag. 1948;28:296–302.
7. MicroscopyU. The source for microscopy education. Introduction to polarized light. https://www.microscopyu.com/techniques/polarized-light/introduction-to-polarized-light. Accessed 21 Jan 2020.
8. Takatsui F, Andrade MF, Neisser MP, Barros LA, Loffredo LC. CIE *L** *a** *b**: comparison of digital images obtained photographically by manual and automatic modes. Braz Oral Res. 2012;26:578–83. https://doi.org/10.1590/s1806-83242012005000025.
9. Hein S, Zangl M. The use of standardized grey reference card in dental photography to correct the effects of five commonly used diffusers on the color of 40 extracted human teeth. Int J Esthet Dent. 2016;11(2):246–59.
10. Sampaio CS, Atria PJ, Hirata R, Jorquera G. Variability of color matching with different digital photography techniques and a gray reference card. J Prosthet Dent. 2018;121(2):333–9. https://doi.org/10.1016/j.prosdent.2018.03.009.
11. Hein S, Tapia J, Bazos P. eLABor_aid: a new approach to digital shade management. Int J Esthet Dent. 2017;12(2):186–202.
12. Jorquera GJ, Atria PJ, Galán M, Feureisen J, Imbarak M, Kernitsky J, Cacciuttolo F, Hirata R, Sampaio CS. A comparison of ceramic crown color difference between different shade selection methods: visual, digital camera, and smartphone. J Prosthet Dent. 2021; https://doi.org/10.1016/j.prosdent.2020.07.029.
13. Bartholin E. Experimenta crystalli islandici disdiaclastici quibus mira & insolita refractio detegitur. Munich: The Bavarian State Library; 1669.
14. Schoppmeier CM, Derman SHM, Noack MJ, Wicht MJ. Power bleaching enhances resin infiltration masking effect of dental fluorosis. A randomized clinical trial. J Dent. 2018;79:77–84. https://doi.org/10.1016/j.jdent.2018.10.005.

6 Bleaching Procedures

Vinícius Salgado

6.1 Tooth Discoloration Etiology

The color of teeth is determined by a combination of intrinsic color and the presence of any extrinsic colored stain that may form on the tooth surface. The tooth discoloration can be classified according to the origin of stain in intrinsic, extrinsic, or internalized discoloration [1].

Intrinsic tooth color is associated with the light energy interaction with the dental tissues such as reflection, transmission, scattering, and absorption optical phenomena [2]. The enamel is a highly mineralized tissue (about 97%) mainly constituted of colorless hydroxyapatite crystals in needles-shape that form a complex, hierarchical, and organized microstructure. The enamel has a slight white color and higher translucency. The dentin is a protein-rich bone-like biocomposite tissue containing a mineral phase (about 70%) mainly constituted by hydroxyapatite, an organic phase mainly constituted by collagen and water. Its hue varies among yellow, orange, and brown shades with low translucency.

The intrinsic tooth discoloration occurs following a change in tooth structural composition or thickness of the hard dental tissues, altering the light-transmitting properties of tooth structure. The intrinsic tooth discoloration may be related to factors that occur prior to tooth eruption during tooth development as metabolic disorders of *Alkaptonuria*, *congenital erythropoietic porphyria*, *congenital hyperbilirubinemia*, *amelogenesis imperfecta*, *dentinogenesis imperfecta*, molar incisor hypomineralization, other systemic syndromes, and to inherited disorders which involve only the hard tissue forming at the time as tetracycline staining, fluorosis, enamel hypoplasia [2] (Figs. 6.1, 6.2, 6.3, 6.4, 6.5 and 6.6).

However, intrinsic tooth staining can also occur after tooth eruption. First, it is related to physiological aging, which increases tooth color darkness. Due to continuous chemical and mechanical wear of enamel through age, that becomes thinner and more translucent, i.e., the dentin will become more visible. Furthermore, the darkness of tooth color intensifies due to the physiological laying down of secondary dentin,

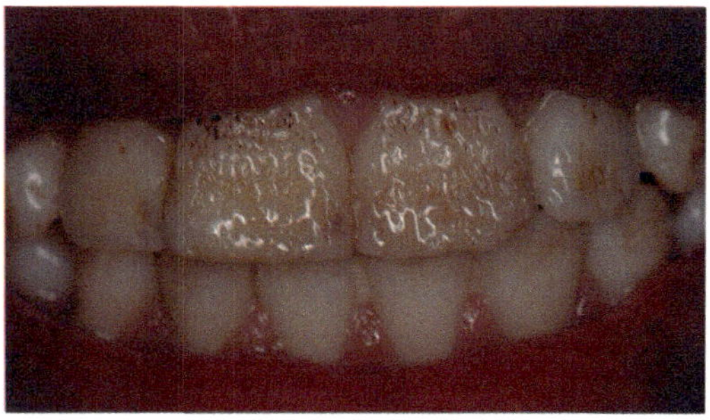

Fig. 6.1 Intrinsic tooth discoloration related to inherited disorders that occur prior to tooth eruption: Amelogenesis imperfecta (Photography courtesy of Dr. Dayane Oliveira et al.)

V. Salgado (✉)
Private Practice, Rio de Janeiro, RJ, Brazil

D. Oliveira (ed.), *Color Science and Shade Selection in Operative Dentistry*,
https://doi.org/10.1007/978-3-030-99173-9_6

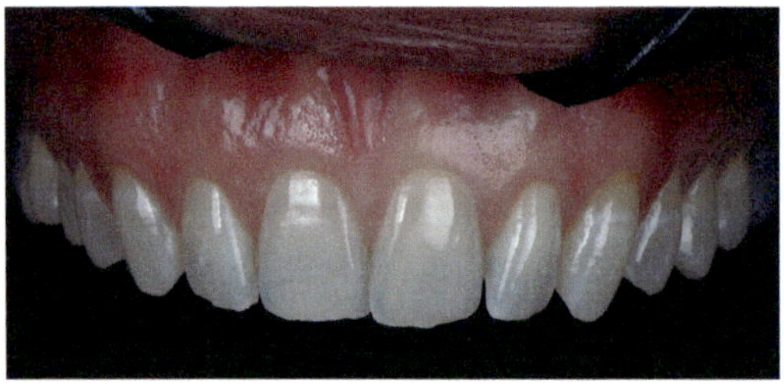

Fig. 6.2 Intrinsic tooth discoloration related to inherited disorders that occur prior to tooth eruption: mild tetracycline staining

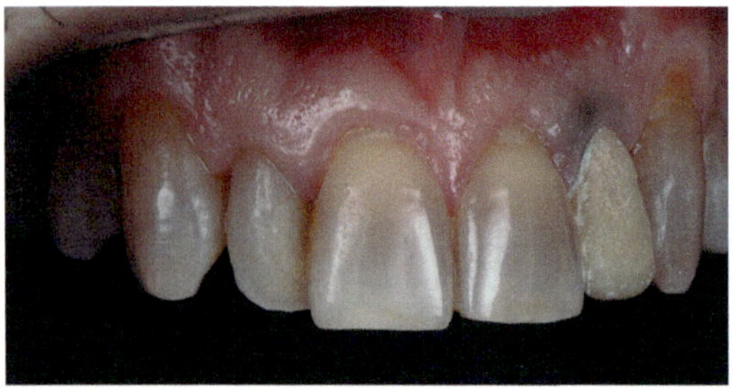

Fig. 6.3 Intrinsic tooth discoloration related to inherited disorders that occur prior to tooth eruption: severe tetracycline staining

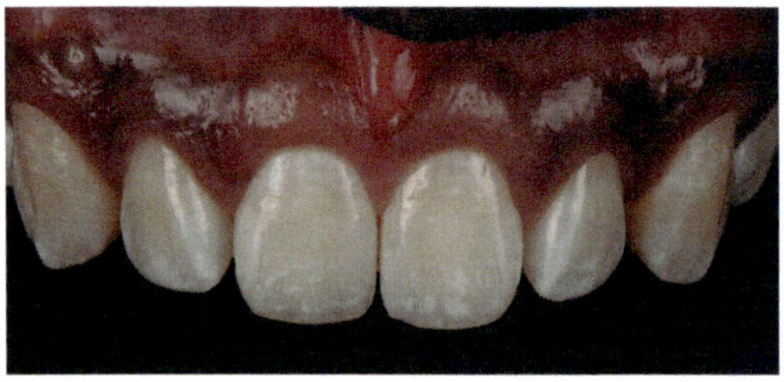

Fig. 6.4 Intrinsic tooth discoloration related to inherited disorders that occur prior to tooth eruption: mild fluorosis staining

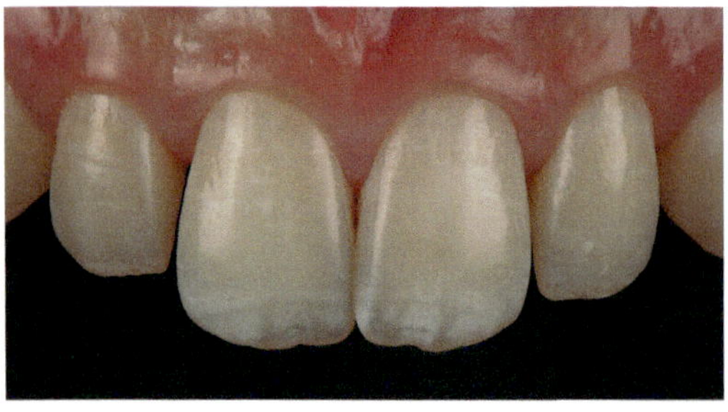

Fig. 6.5 Intrinsic tooth discoloration related to inherited disorders that occur prior to tooth eruption: moderate fluorosis staining

which lead to increased chroma and decreased value of dentin shade [3]. Some inherited disorders that occur after tooth eruption can also leads to intrinsic staining (Figs. 6.7, 6.8, 6.9 and 6.10) as pulpal hemorrhagic products following dental trauma, pulp necrosis, or root resorption [1].

Extrinsic color is associated with the absorption of darker or high-colored compounds,

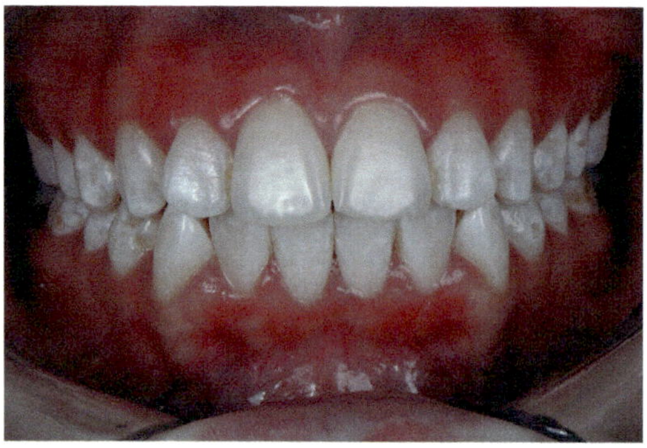

Fig. 6.6 Intrinsic tooth discoloration related to inherited disorders that occur prior to tooth eruption: severe fluorosis staining

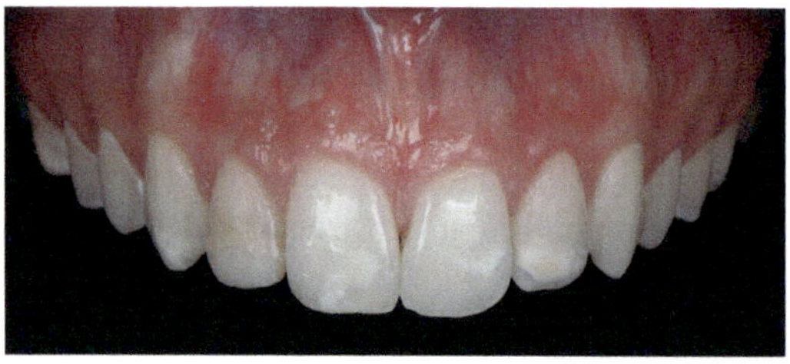

Fig. 6.7 Intrinsic tooth discoloration related to inherited disorders that occur prior to tooth eruption: molar incisor hypomineralization

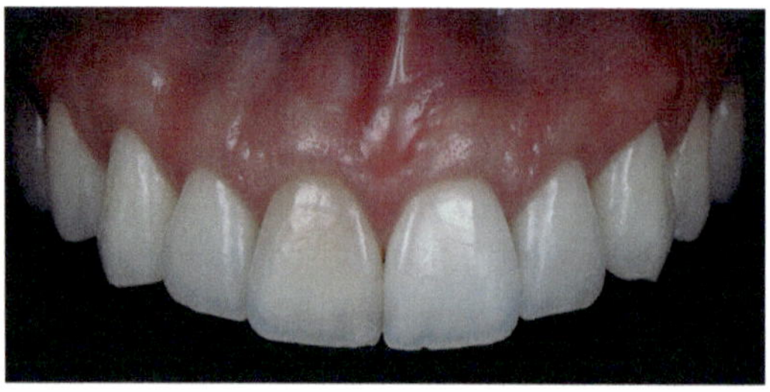

Fig. 6.8 Intrinsic tooth discoloration related to inherited disorders that occur after to tooth eruption: element 11 with history of dental trauma leading to pulp chamber obliteration and darkening aspect

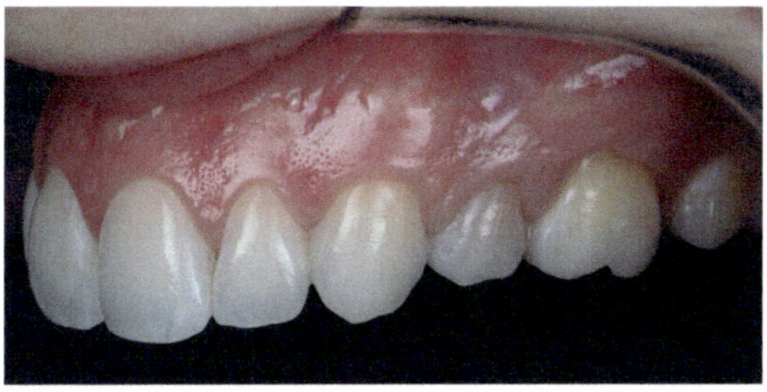

Fig. 6.9 Intrinsic tooth discoloration related to inherited disorders that occur after to tooth eruption: element 25 with pulp necrosis which leads to a gray staining

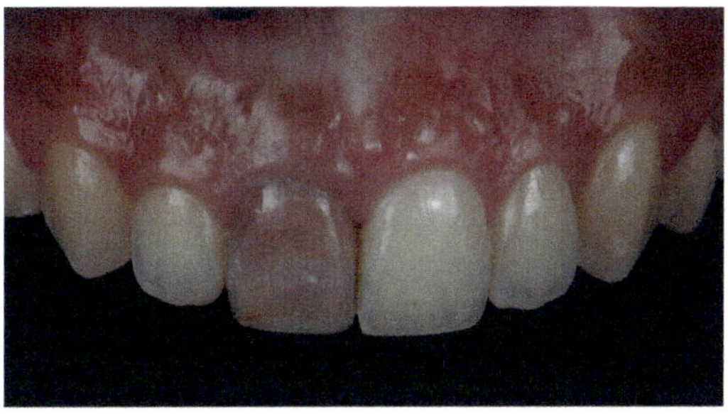

Fig. 6.10 Intrinsic tooth discoloration related to inherited disorders that occur after to tooth eruption: element 11 with history of dental trauma. Situation after 5 years of endodontic treatment and patient's report of progressively darkening intensification. Brownish staining due pulp hemorragic products oxidation

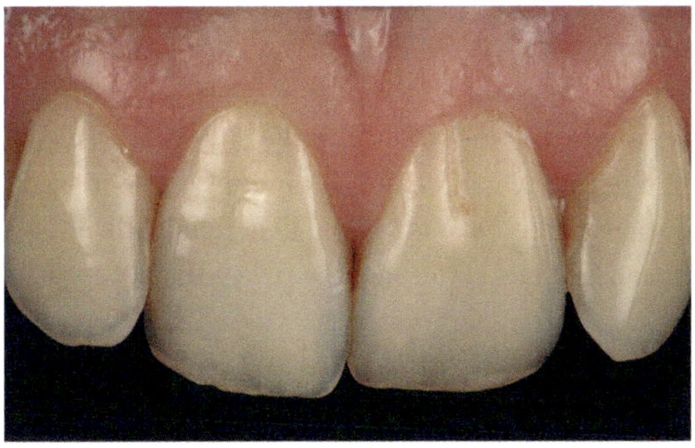

Fig. 6.11 Extrinsic tooth discoloration related to deposition of chromogens onto the dental surface

named chromogens by the pellicle coating (a salivary protein film) and to their deposition onto the enamel surface (Figs. 6.11 and 6.12). There are two different chromogen types: (1) large organic molecules that have conjugated double bonds in their chemical structure and (2) metal-containing molecules. The dental extrinsic staining is influenced by inadequate tooth brushing, dietary intake of colored food and solutions (e.g., coffee, tea, cola soda, and red wine), exposure to nicotine and other tobacco products, and use of cationic agents such chlorhexidine and metal salts (e.g. tin and iron) [1]. Inorganic chromophores are colored transition metal ions of iron, copper, manganese, or tin. In the form of metal complexes, organic and inorganic chromophores may also be present in combination, e.g., in hemoglobin, where a colored porphyrin ligand is combined with a colored iron [4].

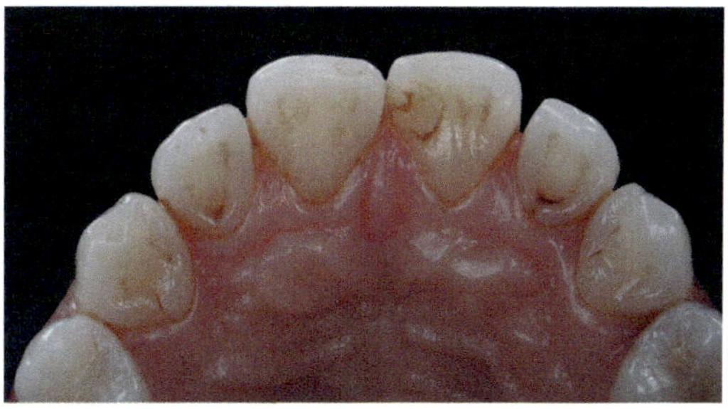

Fig. 6.12 Extrinsic tooth discoloration related to deposition of chromogens onto the dental surface

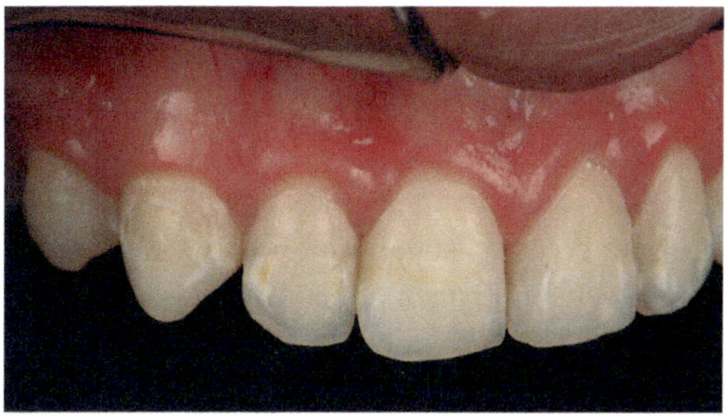

Fig. 6.13 Internalized discoloration related to extrinsic stain incorporation within the tooth structure due enamel porous surface by dental caries

The internalized discoloration is the extrinsic stain incorporation within the tooth structure, mainly those associated with dietary and tobacco products chromogens. It becomes more evident in enamel defects (i.e., fluorosis, dental caries, and enamel cracks, hypoplasia, and hypocalcification) and in the porous surface of exposed dentin [5–7] (Fig. 6.13).

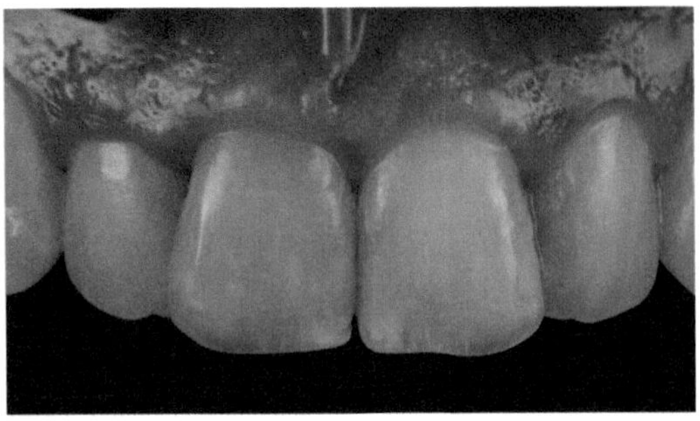

Fig. 6.14 Intrinsic tooth discoloration related to inherited disorders that occur after to tooth eruption: element 11 with history of dental trauma. Situation after 3 years of endodontic treatment and patient's report of progressively darkening intensification. Yellowish/orangewish staining due endodontic products oxidation

Some restorative materials may have an effect on tooth color, as some used for root canal treatment as eugenol, phenolic compounds, and polyantibiotic pastes, which contain pigments that lead to dentin discoloration (Fig. 6.14). Some amalgam alloys may lead to dark grey discoloration of dentin due to tin and mercury penetration in dentinal tubules [8].

6.2 Tooth Whitening Techniques

Tooth whitening can be described as any process that increases teeth lightness. It can be achieved by mechanical or chemical removal of darker or high-colored compounds which are accumulated on the surface or inside the dental tissues.

The extrinsic stain related to the acquired pellicle on the tooth surface can be removed by tooth brushing and flossing while those adhered to the enamel, i.e., dental calculus, by abrasive and polishing action of professional dental prophylaxis. The control of extrinsic stains formation can be made using daily dentifrice containing abrasive agents, which increases the stain cleaning, or/and chemical agents as phosphate salts and enzymes, which prevent their aggregation into the surface [9].

6.2.1 Bleaching Agents

Bleaching is defined as a discoloration process that can occur in a solution or surface. The dental bleaching process may be defined as the chemical degradation of the enamel and dentin chromogens by reactive molecules as peroxides or sodium hypochlorite. Currently available peroxide-containing materials for tooth whitening include professionally dispensed products for supervised at-home use by patients, in-office products use by professionals, and over-the-counter products for sale directly to patients [10].

6.2.1.1 Hydrogen Peroxide

In general, the bleaching mechanism with peroxides is considered to be oxidation, although the process is not well understood. *Hydrogen peroxide* is a highly reactive molecule with low molecular weight. It diffuses into and through the enamel to reach the enamel dentine junction and dentin regions, reacting with the organic molecules, oxidizing the double bonds in conjugated chains and cleaving them. The reaction process forms a number of different active oxygen species depending on conditions, including temperature, pH, light activation, and presence of transition metals [10, 11].

6.2.1.2 Carbamide Peroxide

The *carbamide peroxide* is a chemical adduct of urea and hydrogen peroxide, which, when in contact with water or saliva, disassociates back into hydrogen peroxide and urea. A carbamide peroxide at 10% yields close to 3–3.6% of hydrogen peroxide and 6.4–7% of urea [10]. While hydrogen peroxide can be considered its active ingredient, urea may provide some beneficial side effects because it tends to raise the pH of the solution.

6.2.1.3 Sodium Perborate

The *sodium perborate* is an oxidizing agent available as a powder. It is stable when dry, but it breaks down, which when in contact with water to form sodium metaborate, hydrogen peroxide, and nascent oxygen. Sodium perborate is easier to control, and it considers safer than concentrated hydrogen peroxide solutions [12].

6.2.1.4 Alternative Molecules

The *sodium percarbonate* is an alternative hydrogen peroxide source. It is used in a silicone polymer containing paint-on gel that is applied onto the tooth surface, forming a durable pellicle for overnight bleaching [13]. Alternative tooth bleaching molecules were proposed as *sodium chlorite*, *peroxymonosulphate*, *metal catalysts associated with peroxides* and *oxidoreductase enzymes,* but their efficacy and long-term acceptability require further investigations [10].

6.2.2 Vital Tooth Whitening

There are a number of methods and approaches that have been described in the literature for bleaching of vital teeth with variation in different agents, concentrations, times of applications, product formats, application modes, and light activation [11]. Vital teeth can be bleached at home using dentist-dispensed or over-the-counter products, and/or in the dental office by professional application products.

6.2.2.1 Dentist-Monitored At-Home Bleaching

The original concept of *at-home bleaching* was introduced in 1989 by Haywood and Heymann, also called *nightguard bleaching* [14]. It consists of 10% carbamide peroxide gel use in a customized tray for at least 2 weeks with the supervision and guidance of a dentist [14, 15]. Depending on the tooth darkness and staining type, results are generally seen 2–3 weeks, and the final outcome may be complete in 5–6 weeks. Later products have offered gel concentrations of 1–10% of hydrogen peroxide and 10–22% of carbamide peroxide.

Individual custom-fitted bleaching trays can be made with 0.5–1.0 mm silicon sheets in a heat and vacuum tray-forming machine over plaster models. After cooling, the trays should be cut 2 mm above the gingival margins. Then, it should be tested in the mouth to check their adaption and if any sharp edges bother the tongue and cheeks. The dentist must demonstrate to the patient the application of the whitening gel on the internal facial surface of the tray. Patients should be advised to perform oral hygiene before the bleaching tray application (Figs. 6.15, 6.16, 6.17, 6.18, 6.19, 6.20, 6.21 and 6.22).

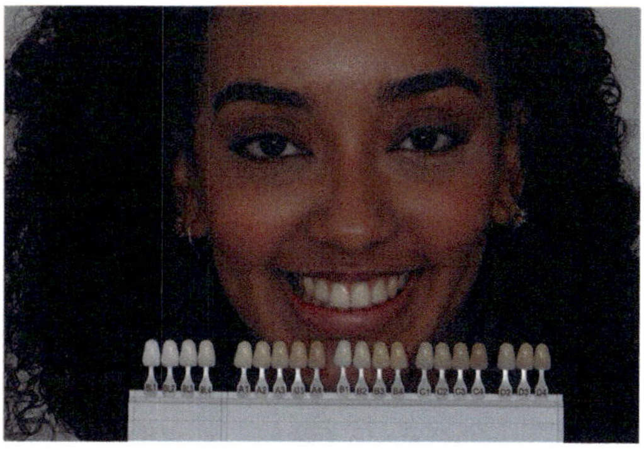

Fig. 6.15 At-home bleaching: initial situation. Face photography

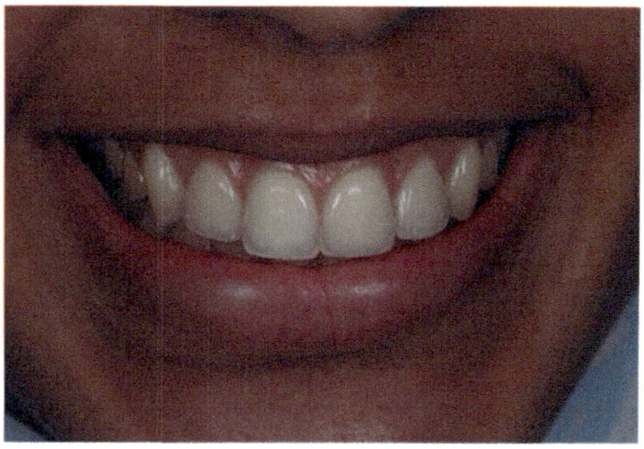

Fig. 6.16 At-home bleaching: initial situation. Smile photography

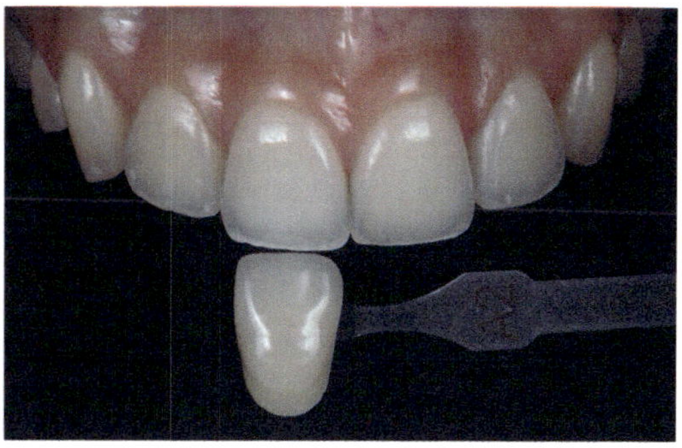

Fig. 6.17 At-home bleaching: initial situation. Intraoral photography

The vital teeth tooth whitening efficacy is determined mainly by the bleaching agent concentration and application period, among several other factors. Basically, the higher the concentration, the faster the whitening effect. However, low concentrations of hydrogen or carbamide

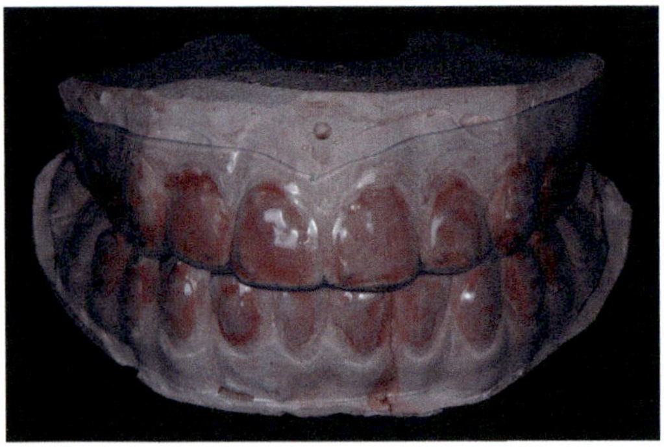

Fig. 6.18 At-home bleaching: individual custom-fitted bleaching trays over plaster models

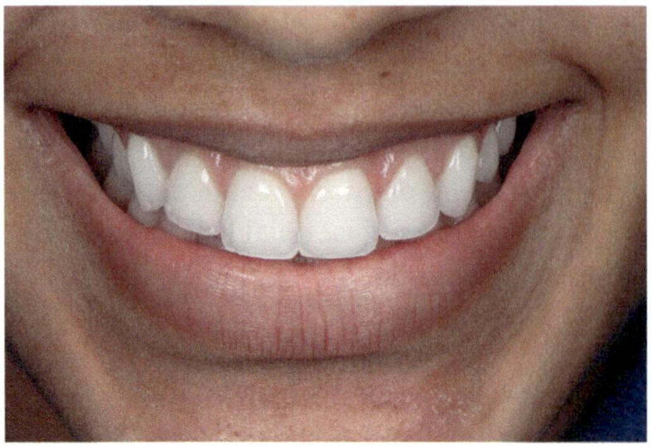

Fig. 6.21 At-home bleaching: final situation. Smile photography

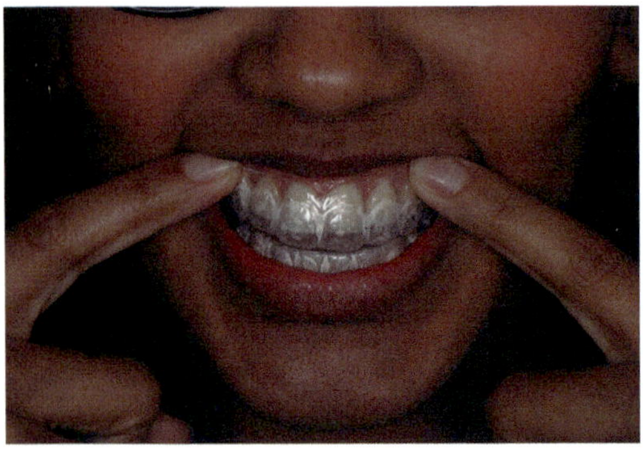

Fig. 6.19 At-home bleaching: bleaching trays test to check their adaption and if any sharp edges bother the tongue and cheeks

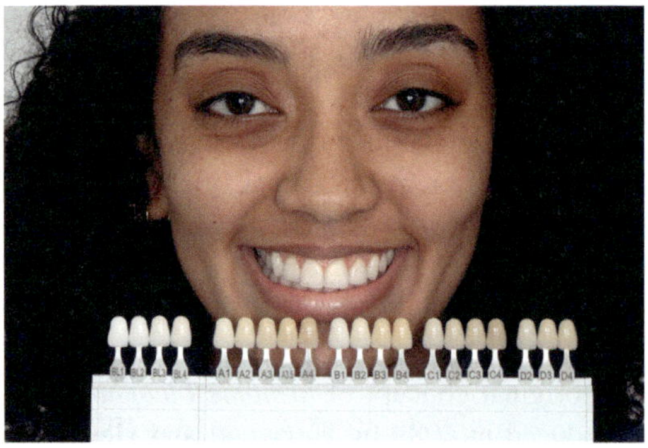

Fig. 6.22 At-home bleaching: final situation. Face photography

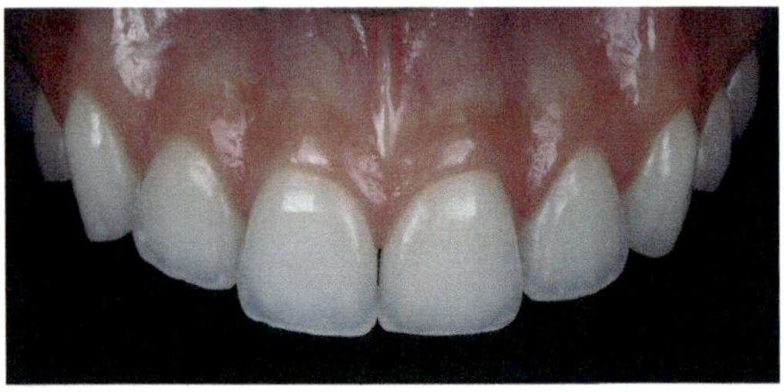

Fig. 6.20 At-home bleaching: final situation. Intraoral photography

peroxides can lead to the same efficacy with an extension of the treatment period [16, 17]. Also, the type of intrinsic stain and initial tooth color plays a significant part in the tooth whitening outcome. The efficacy of the at-home bleaching technique has been demonstrated successful for approximately 91% of non-tetracycline staining teeth but less successful with tetracycline discolored teeth. Tetracycline-stained teeth are the least responsive to bleaching; depending on the severity of the stain, mild to moderate stains tend to respond to extended bleaching regimes of 2–6 months, while severe stains are difficult to bleach. The darker the initial color, the longer the treatment time [18].

Adhering to a white diet during the process (e.g., avoid colorful food and beverages) of tooth whitening does not impair the esthetic outcome [19]. However, patients should be notified to avoid the consumption of citrus food or acidic drinks (due to their low pH) to decrease the risk of teeth hypersensitivity.

In some countries like in the USA, there are mass-market products directly available to the general public. These products contain low concentrations of peroxide agents (e.g., 3–6% hydrogen peroxide) that are self-applied to teeth in different forms as gum shields, strips, and paint-on gels. Usually, it requires two daily applications by 2 weeks approximately [10, 13, 20].

6.2.2.2 In-Office Bleaching of Vital Teeth

High concentrations of peroxide agents are used for professional in-office bleaching of vital teeth, also known as *power bleaching*. It can result in significant whitening after just one professional application, but it requires multiple appointments for optimum whitening results. For vital teeth, hydrogen peroxide at 25–35%, or carbamide peroxide at 35%, are used in short periods of time, between 20 and 40 min of application (Figs. 6.23, 6.24, 6.25, 6.26, 6.27, 6.28, 6.29 and 6.30).

Before application of bleaching gel, the soft tissues should be protected. First, it should be selected an effective lip retractor that also protects the tongue and cheeks from contact with the bleaching gel. A sliced sucker or bite block can be used to restrain dental occlusion and retract the tongue if the lip retractor cannot promote this (Figs. 6.31 and 6.32). Then, a gingival barrier must be applied on the gingival margins of the dental crowns and then photoactivated. Therefore, the bleaching agent should be applied to the teeth labial surface, according to the manufacturer's instructions.

The bleaching gels may be further activated by light, despite the irrelevance of light activation in

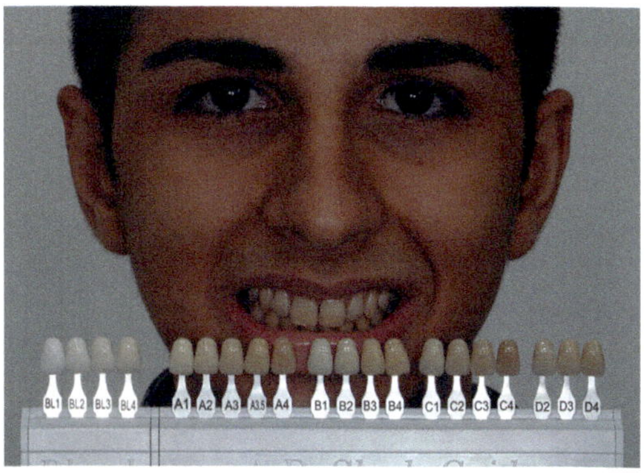

Fig. 6.23 In-office bleaching: initial situation. Face photography

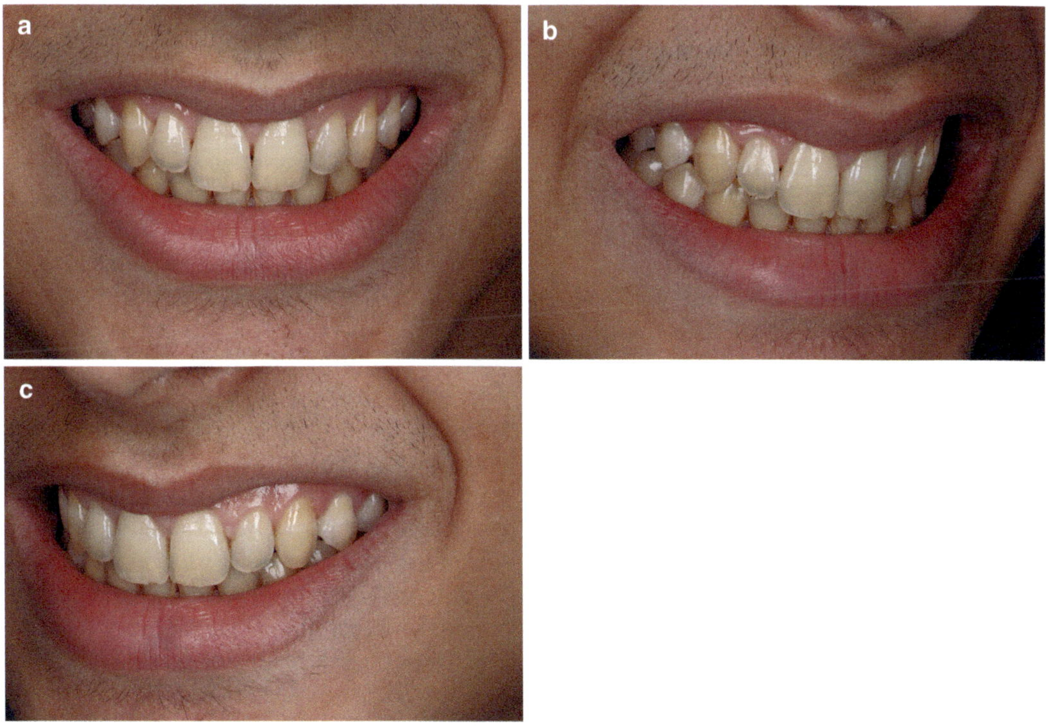

Fig. 6.24 In-office bleaching: initial situation. Smile photography—front (**a**), right (**b**), and left (**c**)

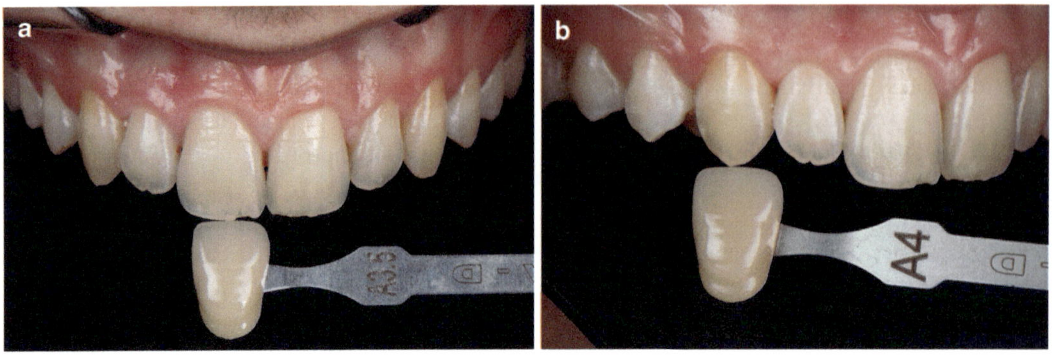

Fig. 6.25 In-office bleaching: initial situation. Intraoral photography and color measurement for incisors (**a**) and canines (**b**)

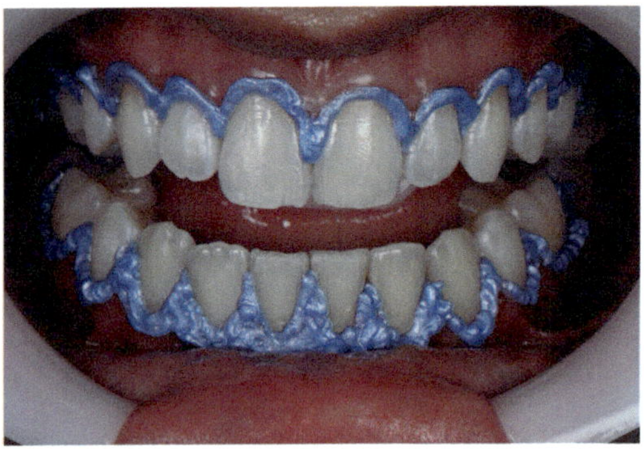

Fig. 6.26 In-office bleaching: soft tissues protection with tongue, chicks, and lips retractor and gingival barrier application

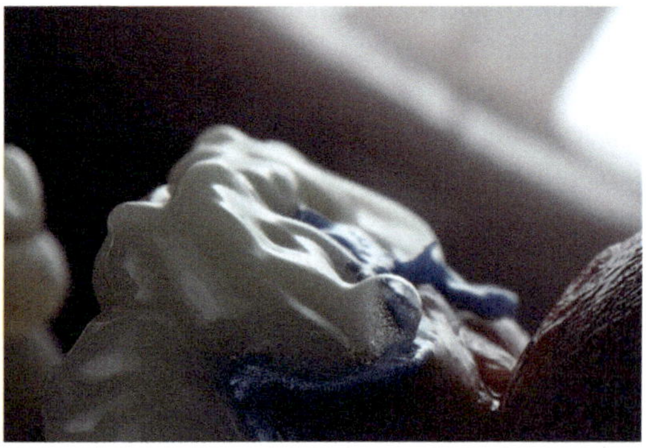

Fig. 6.28 In-office bleaching: bubble formation into the bleaching gel during bleaching reaction

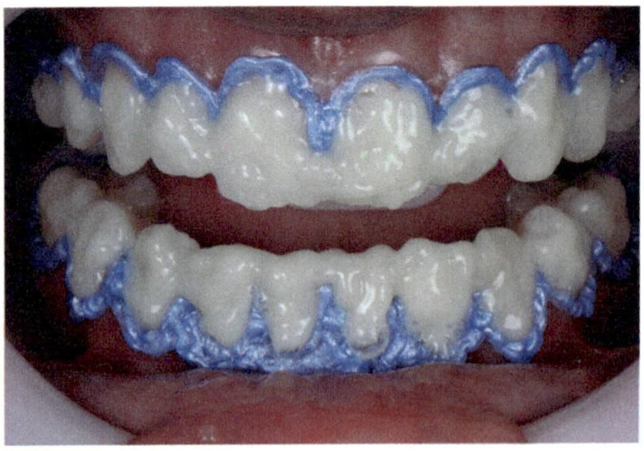

Fig. 6.27 In-office bleaching: application of in-office peroxide gel over teeth surface

the efficacy of tooth whitening. Also, the combination of in-office and at-home bleaching techniques can increase the rate of bleaching in shorter periods of time. However, the bleaching efficacy is not dependent on the technique used [21].

6.2.3 Non-Vital Tooth Whitening

6.2.3.1 Walking Bleaching

The intracoronal or internal bleaching, also known as the *walking bleaching technique,* was introduced in 1967 by Nutting and Poe [22] and is probably the most popular option for bleaching non-vital teeth. Originally, this technique involves filling the pulp chamber with a mixture of 20–30% hydrogen peroxide and sodium perborate, which needs to be reapplied every 2–7 days [15]. However, other peroxide agents can be used as hydrogen peroxide (up to 35%), carbamide peroxide (16–37%), or sodium perborate alone (i.e., mixed with water) [12].

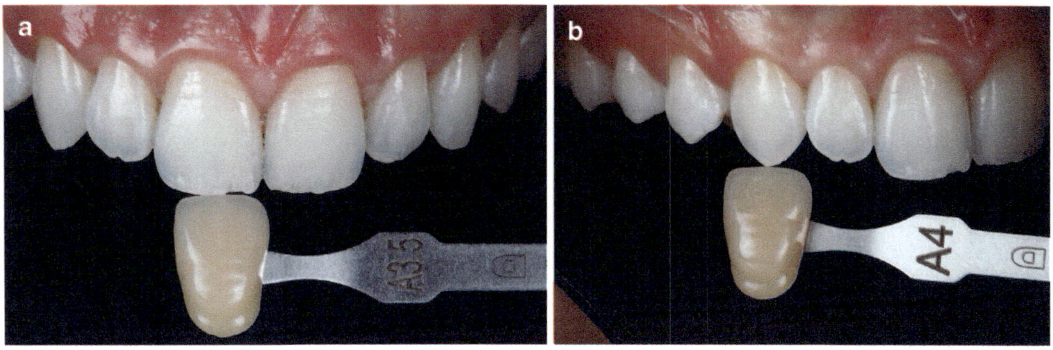

Fig. 6.29 In-office bleaching: final situation after three appointments: intraoral photography and color measurement for incisors (**a**) and canines (**b**)

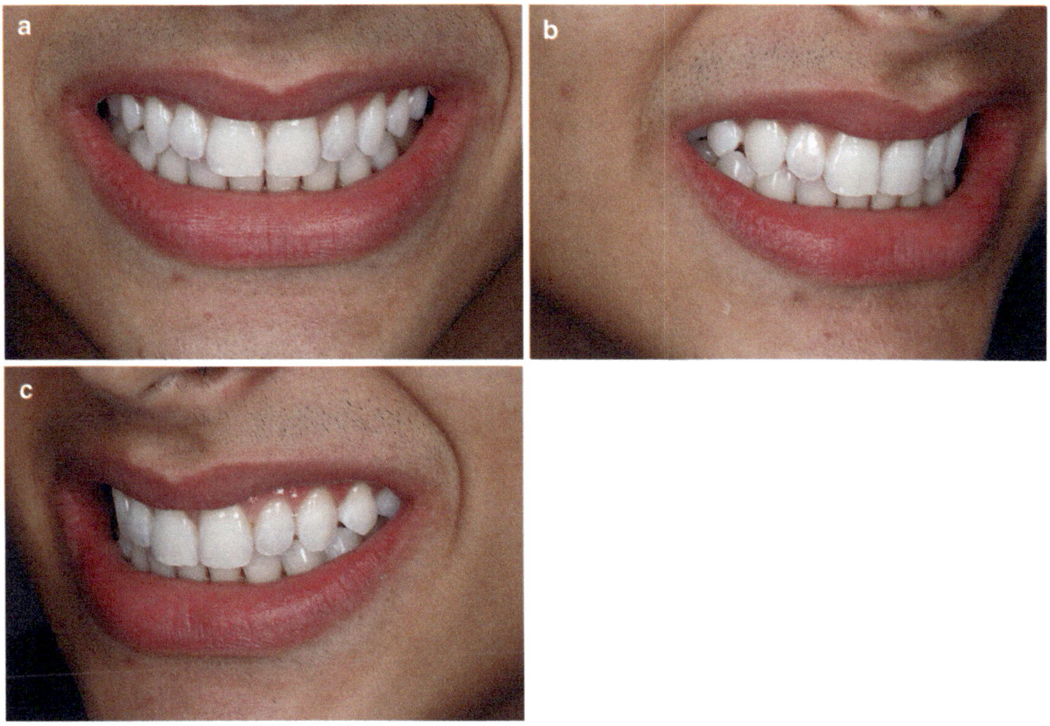

Fig. 6.30 In-office bleaching: final situation: Smile photography—front (**a**), right (**b**), and left (**c**)

After the access to the pulp chamber of endodontic treated teeth, the sealing material should be removed close to 3 mm in an apical direction beyond the clinical crown height to create a space for cervical sealing and exposes the dentinal tubules directed towards the cervical region of the tooth (Figs. 6.9, 6.32, 6.33, 6.34, 6.35, 6.36, 6.37 and 6.38). Then, a 2 mm base of glass-ionomer cement should be applied to protect the endodontic sealing material. Therefore, the bleaching agent is placed into the pulp chamber, cover with a cotton pellet, and then with a provisory restorative material.

The lower the bleaching agent pH, the higher the risk of external cervical root resorption. Although the isolated use of sodium perborate may be a slower process, it is potentially less destructive to the tooth due to its alkaline pH and hence safer.

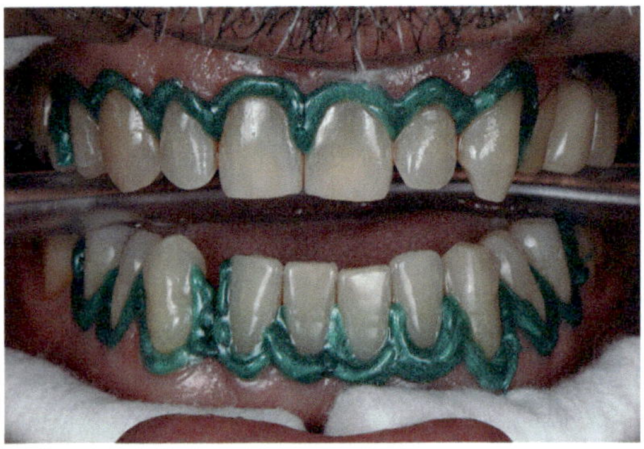

Fig. 6.31 Use of sliced sucker as tongue retractor and to restrain dental occlusion

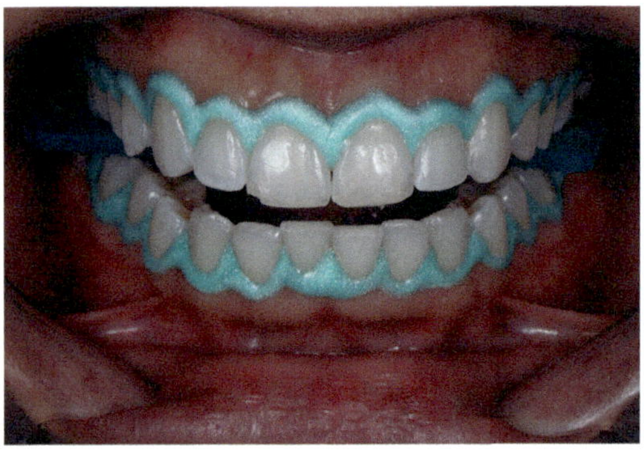

Fig. 6.32 Use of bite block as tongue retractor and to restrain dental occlusion

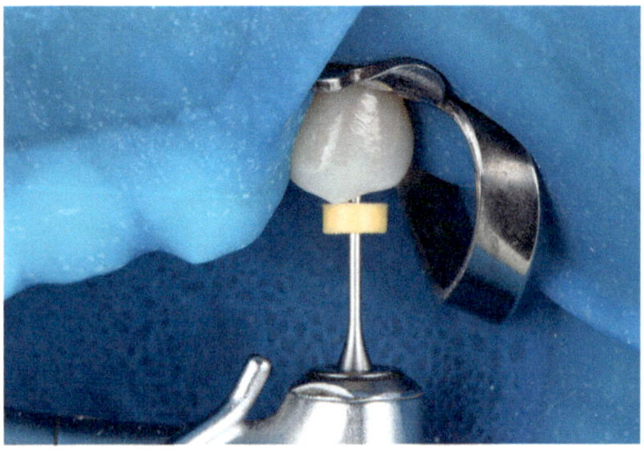

Fig. 6.33 Non-vital bleaching: after endodontic treatment, removal of endodontic sealing material close to 3 mm in an apical direction beyond the clinical crown height to create a space for cervical sealing and exposes the dentinal tubules directed towards the cervical region of the tooth

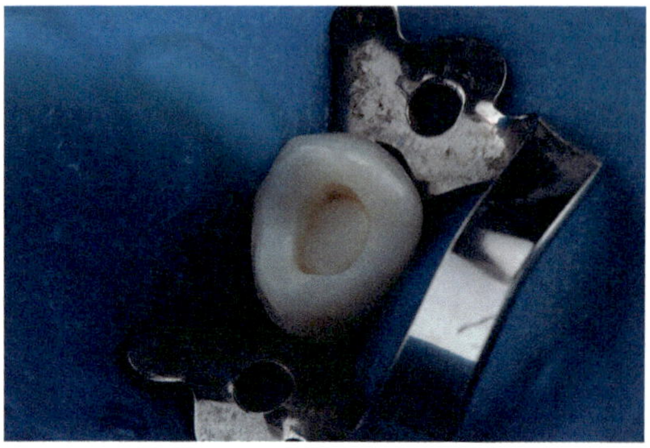

Fig. 6.34 Non-vital bleaching: protection of endodontic sealing material with a 2 mm base of glass-ionomer cement

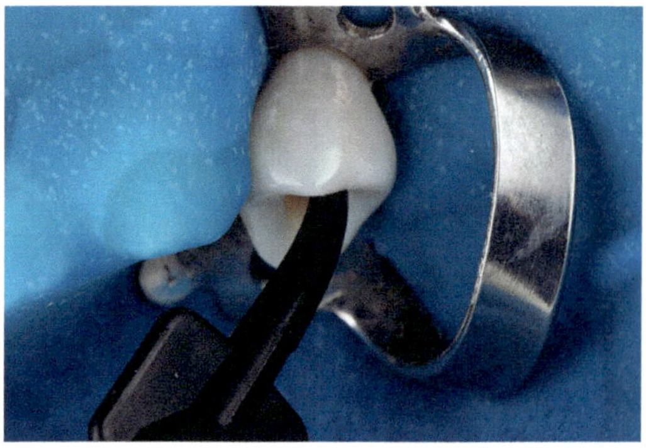

Fig. 6.35 Non-vital bleaching: application of bleaching gel

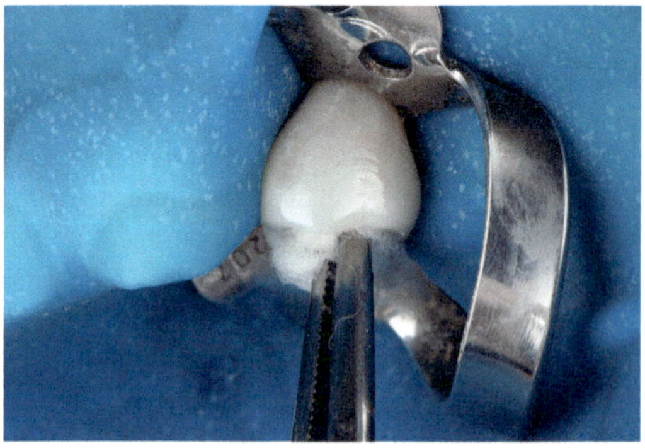

Fig. 6.36 Non-vital bleaching: covering the bleaching gel with a cotton pellet

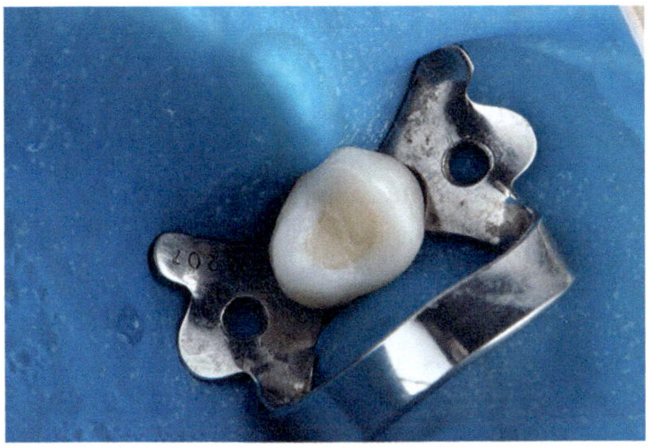

Fig. 6.37 Non-vital bleaching: provisional restoration with provisional direct composite

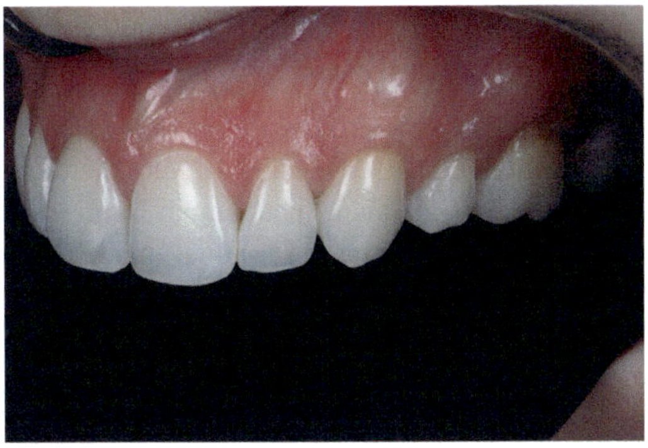

Fig. 6.38 Non-vital bleaching: final situation after 2 weeks of walking bleaching

After the internal bleaching end, the bleaching agent should be removed from the pulp chamber with an extended water flush. Then, the pulp chamber must be provisionally filled with a paste of calcium hydroxide and water in order to render the pH alkaline in the tooth cervical region [23].

6.2.3.2 In-office Internal Bleaching

The *in-office internal bleaching* is considered an alternative treatment for non-vital teeth bleaching. It involves the application of 30–40% hydrogen peroxide inside the pulp chamber and over the external surface of the crown for 20–40 min. In the past, a heating instrument was used to accelerate the process, but this is strongly inadvisable due to the external root cervical resorption increased risk [24].

6.3 Color Measurement for Bleaching Procedures

6.3.1 Patients' Whiteness Perception

The dental color is a frequent concern for patients and is associated with an increased desire for esthetical dental treatments. Psychophysical studies indicate that whitened teeth lead to positive judgements of personality traits such as social competence and appeal, intellectual ability, and relationship satisfaction [25]. The color and overall visual aspect of teeth is a complex phenomenon influenced by several factors as lighting conditions, translucency, opacity, fluorescence, opalescence, iridescence, tooth surface, light scattering, gloss, and human visual system [26]. The teeth whiteness perception by the patients is greatly influenced by the color of their gums, lips, and skin [27, 28]. The darker the color of the tissues around the teeth, the higher the effect of lighter teeth perception. Due to the lower contrast effect, whiter-skinned patients may report less satisfaction with the tooth whitening outcome.

Data from literature indicate that the perception that very white teeth are beautiful significantly decreased with the increase of age group, as well as younger patients expressed a greater preference for white teeth than older patients [29]. Despite the fact that similar expectations with tooth whitening could exist among the different age groups, the standard esthetic preferences are personal. Some patients may seek to have the whitest teeth color possible regardless of their age.

6.3.2 Color Measurement Techniques

As previously mentioned in Chap. 3, there are two different ways to evaluate the color of the teeth, objectively or subjectively. The objective method is based on instrumental color measurements; while the subjective method consists of the visual comparison between teeth and shade guides [30]. The tooth whitening effect can be evaluated both visually and instrumentally. However, the visual method is the most used due its simplicity and reduced cost.

The color of teeth is mainly subjectively measured by the visual comparison method using a tab from paper, colored porcelain, or acrylic resin shade guides [26]. These guides are made of a set of shade tabs intended to cover the range of colors present in human teeth. For tooth whitening monitoring, dental shade guides should be used to follow the color change. Visual evaluation is performed by registering the tab that most closely matches the tooth shade throughout the whitening treatment period.

6.3.2.1 Shade Guides for Tooth Whitening Monitoring

In worldwide clinical practice, the most commonly used dental shade guide is the Vitapan Classical (Vita Zahnfabrik). As mentioned in Chap. 3, the color range of this shade guide is divided into four different hue groups designated by A, B, C, and D letters, representing reddish-brown for A hue, reddish-yellow for B hue, grayish for C hue, and reddish-gray for D hue. For each hue group, there are different tabs differentiated by an Arabic number ranging from 1 to 4, with different chromas and values. The higher the number, the higher chroma and the lower the value. For tooth whitening monitoring, it is recommended to rearrange the tabs according to the value, from the highest (B1) to the lowest (C4) (Fig. 6.39) [31]. Recently, a modification for this shade guide was proposed, adding three new tabs for bleached teeth 0M1, 0M2, and 0M3 [32].

The Bleachedguide 3D-MASTER (Vita Zahnfabrik) is a cross-section of Toothguide 3D-MASTER (Vita Zahnfabrik) with 15 tabs and a linear arrangement from the highest (0M1) to the lowest (5M3) value (Fig. 6.40). It contains 8 original Toothguide 3D-MASTER tabs and 7 interpolated tabs, included to bridge large color differences among middle tab (M2) in different groups. The lightest part of the Bleachedguide 3D-MASTER exhibits subtle color gradation with several tabs lighter than the lightest tab of Vitapan Classical (B1) [33].

There are other value-arranged shade guides exclusively designed for tooth whitening monitoring as the R-20 and R-27 (Vakker Dental) with 20 and 27 tabs, respectively (Fig. 6.41). However, no research data is available in the literature about their use for shade matching in Dentistry.

There are several shade guides made from paper, available to purchase by regular consumers (non-dentists) with different color and whiteness gradations. Its use for tooth whitening monitoring should not be encouraged by clinicians due to the paper perishability, color differences among shade guides due to printing errors, inadequate flat surface of the tabs, or even due to the absence of detachable tabs.

6.3.2.2 Visual Color Measurement

During the tooth whitening monitoring, color measurement should be performed in order to follow the color change. As mentioned in Chap. 3, color from any object, as the tooth and shade guide tab, is directly influenced by illumination.

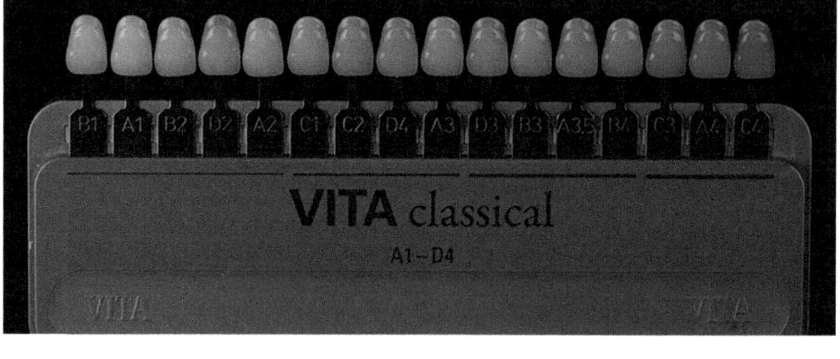

Fig. 6.39 Tooth whitening monitoring: rearrange the Vitapan Classical tabs according to the value, from the highest (B1) to the lowest (C4)

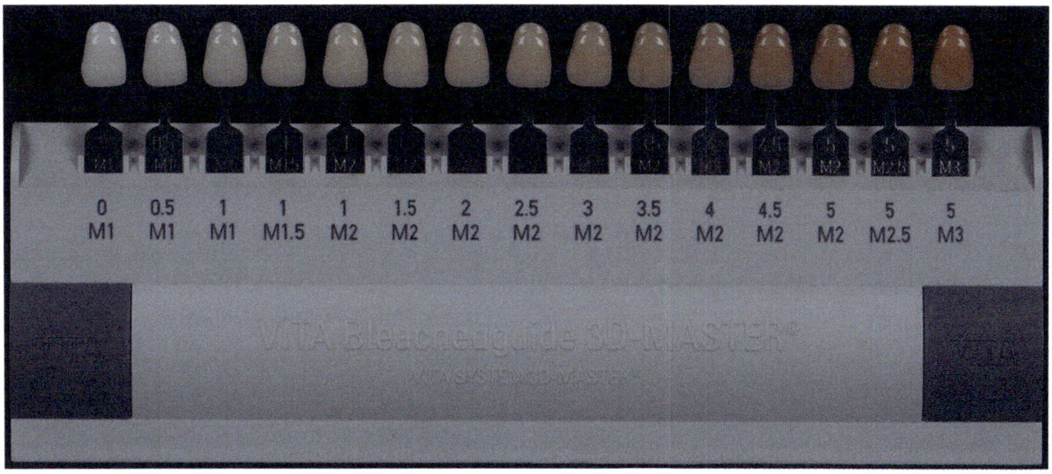

Fig. 6.40 Tooth whitening monitoring: bleachedguide 3D-MASTER shade guide

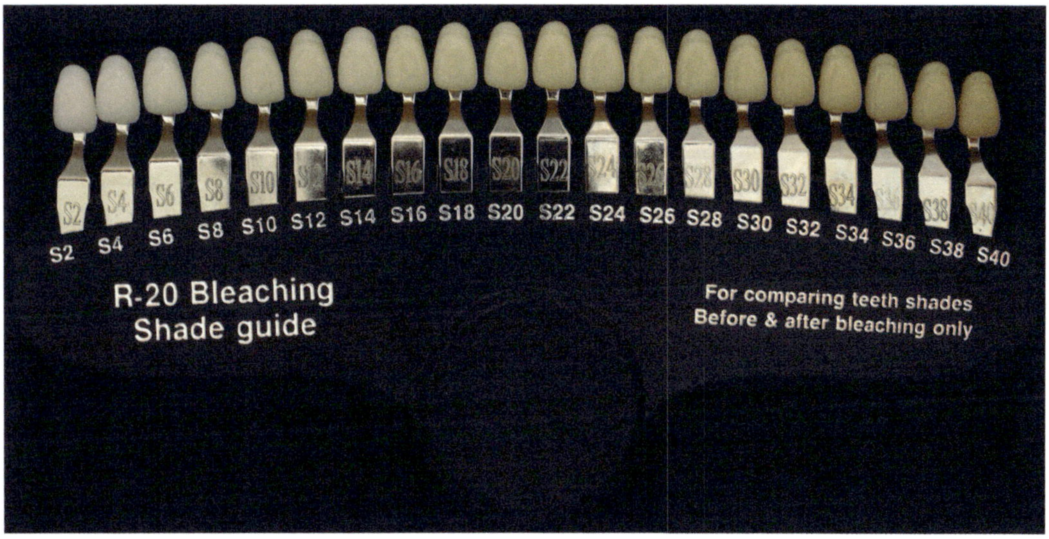

Fig. 6.41 Tooth whitening monitoring: value-arranged R-20 bleaching shade guide

Therefore, it is important to place the tab at an equal level with teeth to get the same amount of illumination.

6.3.2.3 Photographic Register

Taking photographs in the beginning and during the curse of tooth whitening treatment is strongly recommended due to different reasons. Sometimes, patients may be demotivated with the treatment due to self-perception of no efficacy. So, beyond registering the color change throughout the whitening period, taking standardized photographs is necessary to show the patient the treatment evolution.

A photographic protocol is suggested for the beginning and for the end of tooth whitening: (1) full-face smiling photo; (2) face smiling photo with dental shade guide placement just below the smile; smile photos in (3) front, (4) right and left (5) sides; (6) and (7) intraoral photos of upper anterior teeth over a black background with the tab placement that most closely matches the actual color of the upper central incisors (6) and upper canines (7).

During the whitening progress monitoring, the same intraoral photos can also be taken i.e., before-after an in-office power bleaching appointment and at each at-home whitening control appointments.

6.4 Considerations to Bleaching Related to Direct Restorative Approaches

The bleaching procedures may negatively affect the marginal seal of restorations in both pre- and post-operative periods. Meticulously clinical examination must be performed before application of peroxide agents. Unsatisfactory restorations need to be repaired or replaced prior to bleaching in order to achieve an optimal seal of the pulp chamber, reducing the risk of adverse effects [34].

Considering the bleaching of restored teeth, the peroxide agents react to the resin-based composite' components and produce color and surface alterations. They increase the elution of unpolymerized monomers, additives, and other organic components oxidation [35, 36]. At the same time, they are increasing the lightness and decreasing the chroma for the natural tooth; they act in the opposite way on the resin-based composite materials, accentuating the color mismatch between the two structures. Therefore, composite restorations in anterior teeth often need to be replaced after the tooth whitening treatment [35].

During the whitening treatment, teeth get an increase in lightness through the process and reach a maximum lightness regardless of the concentration of the agent or contact time used. With the peroxide agent removal, dental rehydration occurs, and the teeth will get a decrease in lightness due to light absorption by water into the dental tissues. So, for restorative approaches after tooth whitening, it is necessary to wait for at least 10 days before measuring the real tooth color [37].

The peroxide agents oxidizing effect alters the organic matrix of enamel and dentin, impairing a strong and stable bond between the composite applied and the superficial etched enamel layer. Moreover, the residual oxygen present in dental tissues after the bleaching process decreases the bond strength to enamel and dentin, because the oxygen inhibits the monomer polymerization that cures via a free-radical mechanism [38, 39]. For this reason, it is recommended to delay at least 1 week after the tooth whitening before placement/replacement of direct restorations in order to the residual oxygen may have sufficient time to leach from the dental hard tissues. Optimal bonding to pre-bleached dental hard tissue could be achieved after a period of about 3 weeks [35].

References

1. Watts A, Addy M. Tooth discolouration and staining: a review of the literature. Br Dent J. 2001;190(6):309–16.
2. Joiner A, Luo W. Tooth colour and whiteness: a review. J Dent. 2017;67S:S3–S10.
3. Algarni AA, Ungar PS, Lippert F, Martínez-Mier EA, Eckert GJ, González-Cabezas C, Hara AT. Trend-analysis of dental hard-tissue conditions as function of tooth age. J Dent. 2018;74:107–12.
4. Epple M, Meyer F, Enax J. A critical review of modern concepts for teeth whitening. Dent J (Basel). 2019;7(3):79.
5. Ardu S, Benbachir N, Stavridakis M, Dietschi D, Krejci I, Feilzer A. A combined chemo-mechanical approach for aesthetic management of superficial enamel defects. Br Dent J. 2009;206(4):205–8.
6. Paris S, Meyer-Lueckel H. Masking of labial enamel white spot lesions by resin infiltration—a clinical report. Quintessence Int. 2009;40(9):713–8.
7. Attal JP, Atlan A, Denis M, Vennat E, Tirlet G. White spots on enamel: treatment protocol by superficial or deep infiltration (part 2). Int Orthod. 2014;12(1):1–31.
8. Calazans FS, Dias KR, Miranda MS. Modified technique for vital bleaching of teeth pigmented by amalgam: a case report. Oper Dent. 2011;36(6):678–82.
9. Joiner A. Whitening toothpastes: a review of the literature. J Dent. 2010;38(Suppl 2):e17–24.
10. Joiner A. The bleaching of teeth: a review of the literature. J Dent. 2006;34(7):412–9.
11. Joiner A. Review of the effects of peroxide on enamel and dentine properties. J Dent. 2007;35(12):889–96.
12. Plotino G, Buono L, Grande NM, Pameijer CH, Somma F. Nonvital tooth bleaching: a review of the literature and clinical procedures. J Endod. 2008;34(4):394–407.
13. Date RF, Yue J, Barlow AP, Bellamy PG, Prendergast MJ, Gerlach RW. Delivery, substantivity and clinical response of a direct application percarbonate tooth whitening film. Am J Dent. 2003;16:3B–8B.

14. Haywood VB, Heymann HO. Nightguard vital bleaching. Quintessence Int. 1989;20:173–6.
15. Haywood VB. History, safety, and effectiveness of current bleaching techniques and applications of the nightguard vital bleaching technique. Quintessence Int. 1992;23(7):471–88.
16. Mokhlis GR, Matis BA, Cochran MA, Eckert GJ. A clinical evaluation of carbamide peroxide and hydrogen peroxide whitening agents during daytime use. J Am Dent Assoc. 2000;131(9):1269–77.
17. Kihn PW, Barnes DM, Romberg E, Peterson K. A clinical evaluation of 10 percent vs. 15 percent carbamide peroxide tooth-whitening agents. J Am Dent Assoc. 2000;131(10):1478–84.
18. Matis BA, Wang Y, Eckert GJ, Cochran MA, Jiang T. Extended bleaching of tetracycline-stained teeth: a 5-year study. Oper Dent. 2006;31(6):643–51.
19. Matis BA, Wang G, Matis JI, Cook NB, Eckert GJ. White diet: is it necessary during tooth whitening? Oper Dent. 2015;40(3):235–40.
20. Matis BA, Cochran M, Wang G, Franco M, Eckert GJ, Carlotti RJ, Bryan C. A clinical evaluation of bleaching using whitening wraps and strips. Oper Dent. 2005;30(5):588–92.
21. Bernardon JK, Sartori N, Ballarin A, Perdigão J, Lopes GC, Baratieri LN. Clinical performance of vital bleaching techniques. Oper Dent. 2010;35(1):3–10.
22. Nutting EB, Poe GS. Chemical bleaching of discolored endodontically treated teeth. Dent Clin N Am. 1967;16:655–62.
23. Bizhang M, Heiden A, Blunck U, Zimmer S, Seemann R, Roulet JF. Intracoronal bleaching of discolored non-vital teeth. Oper Dent. 2003;28(4):334–40.
24. Harrington GW, Natkin E. External resorption associated with bleaching of pulpless teeth. J Endod. 1979;5:344–8.
25. Höfel L, Lange M, Jacobsen T. Beauty and the teeth: perception of tooth color and its influence on the overall judgment of facial attractiveness. Int J Periodontics Restor Dent. 2007;27(4):349–57.
26. Joiner A. Tooth colour: a review of the literature. J Dent. 2004;32(Suppl 1):3–12.
27. Reno EA, Sunberg RJ, Block RP, Bush RD. The influence of lip/gum color on subject perception of tooth color. J Dent Res. 2000;79:381.
28. Sharma V, Punia V, Khandelwal M, Punia S, Lakshmana R. A study of relationship between skin color and tooth shade value in population of Udaipur, Rajasthan. Int J Dent Clin. 2010;2:26–9.
29. Grosofsky A, Adkins S, Bastholm R, Meyer L, Krueger L, Meyer J, Torma P. Tooth color: effects on judgments of attractiveness and age. Percept Mot Skills. 2003;96:43–8.
30. Chu SJ, Trushkowsky RD, Paravina RD. Dental color matching instruments and systems. Review of clinical and research aspects. J Dent. 2010;38(Suppl 2):e2–16.
31. Browning WD. Use of shade guides for color measurement in tooth-bleaching studies. J Esthet Restor Dent. 2003;15(s1):S13–20.
32. Paravina RD. Performance assessment of dental shade guides. J Dent. 2009;37(Suppl 1):e15–20.
33. Paravina RD. New shade guide for tooth whitening monitoring: visual assessment. J Prosthet Dent. 2008;99:178–84.
34. Gokäy O, Yilmaz F, Akin S, Tuncbilek M, Ertan R. Penetration of the pulp chamber by bleaching agents in teeth restored with various restorative materials. J Endod. 2000;26:92–4.
35. Attin T, Hannig C, Wiegand A, Attin R. Effect of bleaching on restorative materials and restorations—a systematic review. Dent Mater. 2004;20(9):852–61.
36. Della Bona A, Pecho OE, Ghinea R, Cardona JC, Paravina RD, Perez MM. Influence of bleaching and aging procedures on color and whiteness of dental composites. Oper Dent. 2019;44(6):648–58.
37. Kihn PW. Vital tooth whitening. Dent Clin N Am. 2007;51(2):319–31.
38. Rueggeberg FA, Margeson DH. The effect of oxygen inhibition on an unfilled/filled composite system. J Dent Res. 1990;69:1652–8.
39. Turkun M, Turkun LS. Effect of nonvital bleaching with 10% carbamide peroxide on sealing ability of resin composite restorations. Int Endod J. 2004;37:52–60.

7 Biomimetics of the Natural Tooth Using Composites

Dayane Oliveira and Vinícius Salgado

7.1 Build-Up Layering Techniques

The current resin-based composites have different degrees of opacity and translucency. It can be nominated according to the areas that should be located (i.e., cervical, body, or incisal) and to tissues that they must reproduce (i.e., dentin or enamel).

The layering of resin-based composite direct restorations for esthetic purposes started with the light-curing technology development. The major part of resin-based composites is VITA-based, i.e., their colors are based on the *Vitapan Classical* (Vita Zahnfabrik) color concept. They are also named in the same way as these shade guide tabs. First by a letter (A, B, C, and D), which represents the hue, and then by an Arabic number, which represents the chroma degree, the higher the number, the higher the chroma. However, other resin-based composite systems are non-VITA-based, i.e., they have other color concept and different nomenclatures.

Nowadays, there are available several resin-based composite systems with different shading and layering concepts with different levels of clinical complexity and reliability [1]. They can be classified according to the proposed number of shade layers for a restoration, from monochromatic to polychromatic restorations. However, the dentist should know that the esthetic success of its direct restorations is dependent of a learning curve with the use of some specific composite and also with the layering technique.

Before the restorative procedure itself, special attention should be paid to the tooth characteristics, which are related to the patient's age, tooth translucency pattern, tooth wear, and other specific characteristics as surface cracks, and opaque spots or lines [1–3].

7.1.1 One-Layer Build-Up Technique

This concept was created together with the introduction of resin-based composites for direct restorations. It is based on the application of just one shade in all extensions of the restoration. Although it is unable to fully reproduce the optical features of dental tissues, it can be effectively used in small classes III or even in temporary restorations.

With the development of different opacity materials, the optical features of resin-based composites get an improvement, and new possibilities have emerged for this concept

D. Oliveira (✉)
Department of Restorative Dental Sciences, College of Dentistry, University of Florida, Gainesville, FL, USA
e-mail: DOliveira@dental.ufl.edu

V. Salgado
Private Practice, Rio de Janeiro, RJ, Brazil

D. Oliveira (ed.), *Color Science and Shade Selection in Operative Dentistry*,
https://doi.org/10.1007/978-3-030-99173-9_7

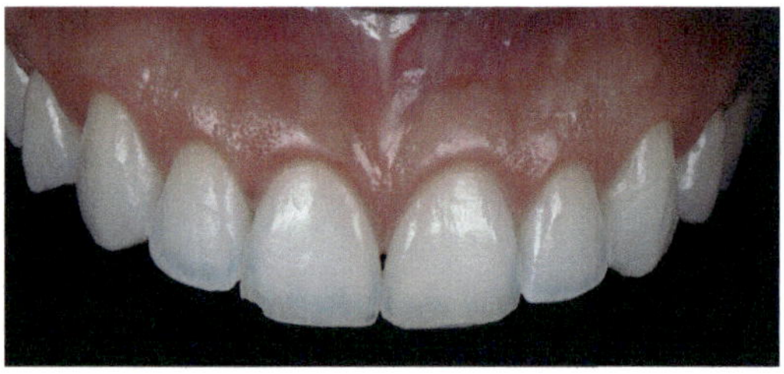

Fig. 7.1 Clinical case of one-layer build-up technique: initial situation

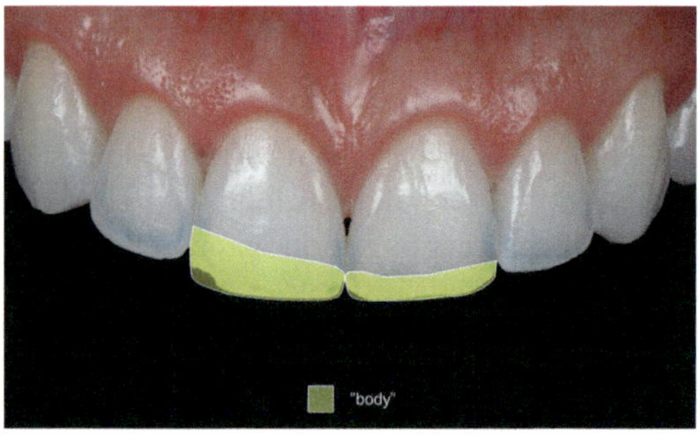

Fig. 7.2 Clinical case of one-layer build-up technique: color stratification planning

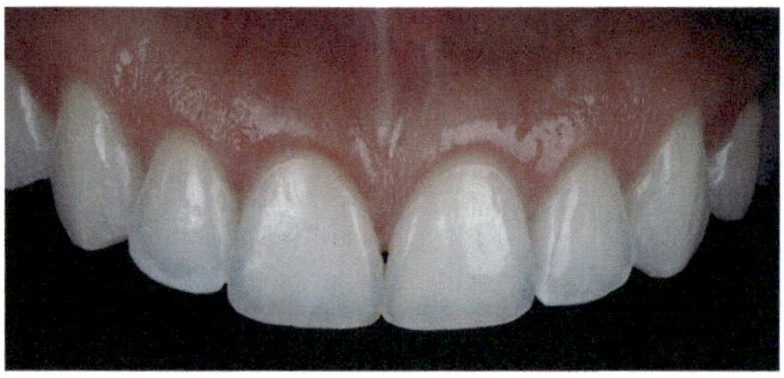

Fig. 7.3 Clinical case of one-layer build-up technique: final situation

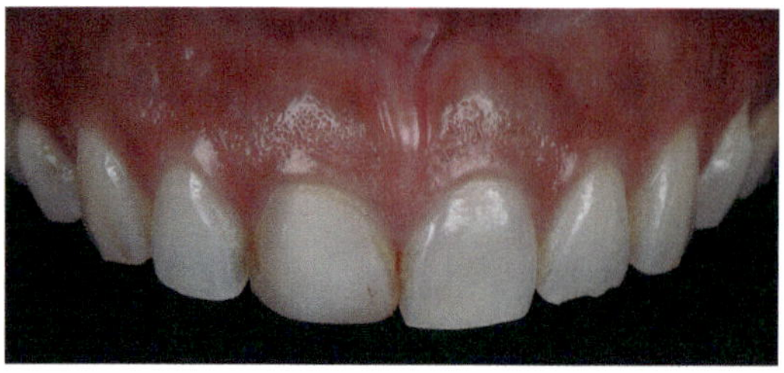

Fig. 7.4 Clinical case of two-layers build-up technique—classical two-layering: initial situation

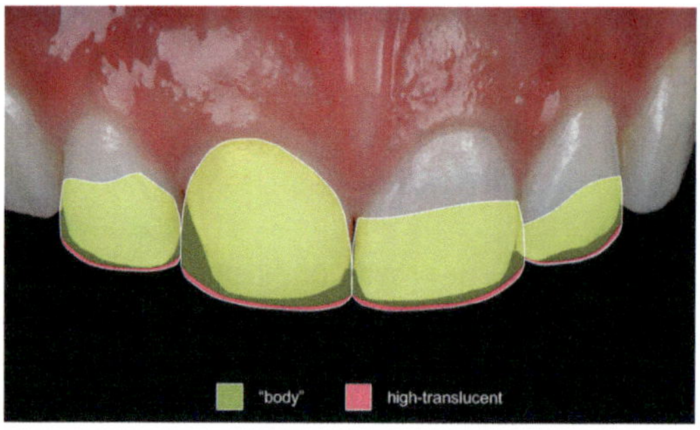

Fig. 7.5 Clinical case of two-layers build-up technique—classical two-layering: color stratification planning

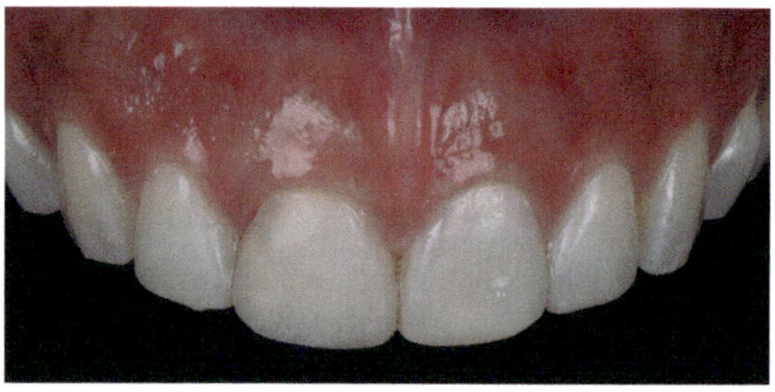

Fig. 7.6 Clinical case of two-layers build-up technique—classical two-layering: final situation

(Figs. 7.1, 7.2 and 7.3). The *Chameleon technique* is based on the monochromatic build-up of the restoration with materials of intermediate opacity, also named as "body" composites, and its blending with the surrounding dental tissues [4].

7.1.2 Two-Layers Build-Up Technique

7.1.2.1 Classical Two-Layering

This concept was developed based on the one-layer build-up in order to improve the esthetic of restorations. It comprises a monochromatic build-up using "body" masses with the addition of high-translucent materials, also named "incisal" or "transparent," in the incisal region in order to reproduce the incisal translucency (Figs. 7.4, 7.5 and 7.6).

7.1.2.2 Natural Two-Layering

This concept relies on the application of two masses, which rather tends to replicate the optical properties of the dental tissues, allowing a spatial

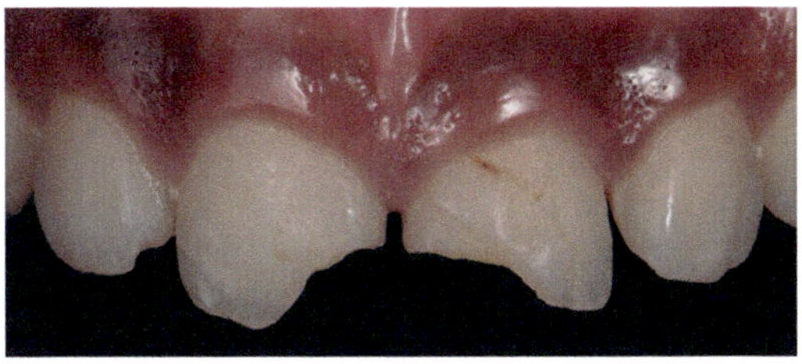

Fig. 7.7 Clinical case of two-layers build-up technique—natural two-layering: initial situation. (*Photography courtesy of Dr. Monique Solon and Dr. Thais Soares*)

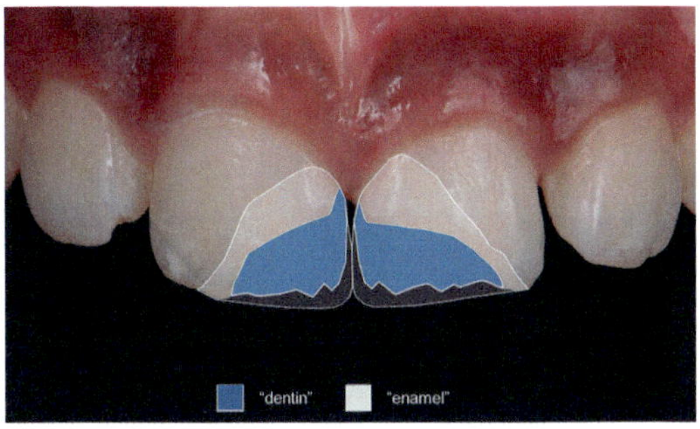

Fig. 7.8 Clinical case of two-layers build-up technique—natural two-layering: color stratification planning. (*Photography courtesy of Dr. Monique Solon and Dr. Thais Soares*)

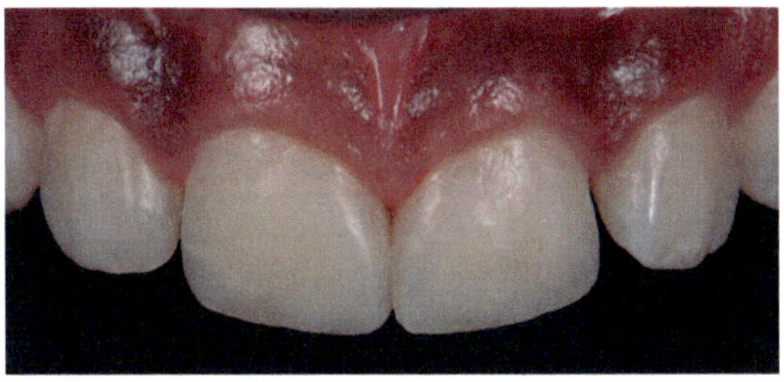

Fig. 7.9 Clinical case of two-layers build-up technique—natural two-layering: final situation. (*Photography courtesy of Dr. Monique Solon and Dr. Thais Soares*)

arrangement that copies the dental structure (Figs. 7.7, 7.8 and 7.9). Opaque masses, named as "dentin" shades, with opacity similar to the natural dentin, are used in the center of the restoration. Covering them are the translucent masses, named "enamel" which may be applied in different aspects to reproduce young, adult, and elderly teeth [5–7].

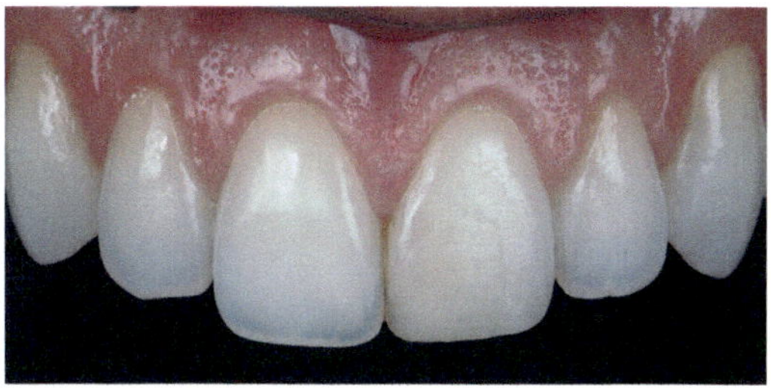

Fig. 7.10 Clinical case of multi-layer build-up technique—classical three-layers: initial situation

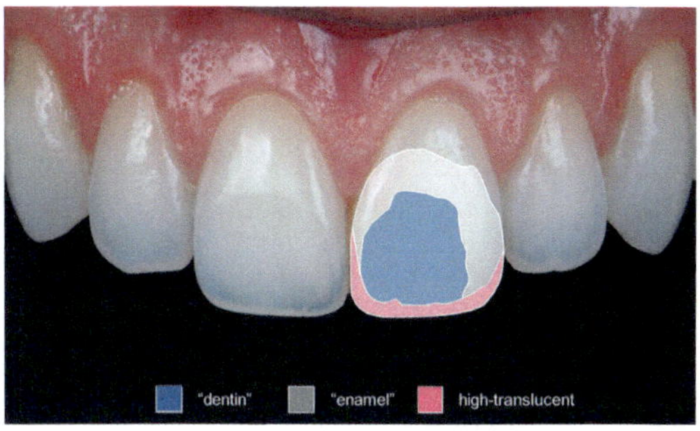

Fig. 7.11 Clinical case of multi-layer build-up technique—classical three-layers: color stratification planning

7.1.3 Multi-Layers Build-Up Technique

7.1.3.1 Classical Three Layers

It comprises a set of three different opacity masses. First, a high-opacity material, named "dentin" shades, are used, followed by a low-opacity material, named "enamel" (or "body" in some restorative systems) shades, and then, by a high-translucent material, named "translucent," "incisal," or "transparent" shades. Different from the natural layering, this concept implies a polychromatic build-up, with opacity and chroma variations from the inside to the outside of the restoration (Figs. 7.10, 7.11 and 7.12).

7.1.3.2 Modern Three Layers

This concept is based on the natural two-layering, but with the addition of "effect" materials to reproduce fine anatomic details, placed between

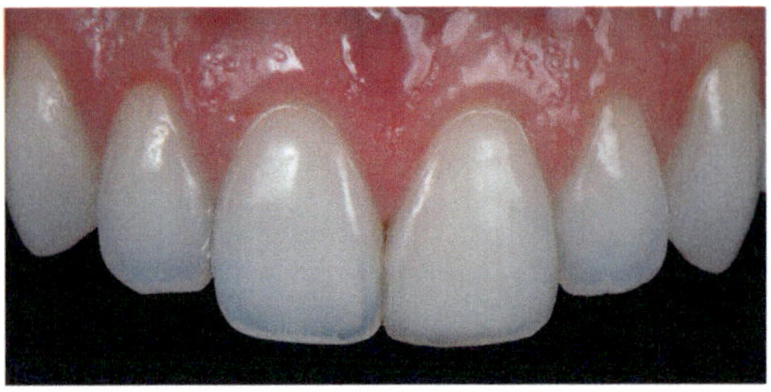

Fig. 7.12 Clinical case of multi-layer build-up technique—classical three-layers: final situation

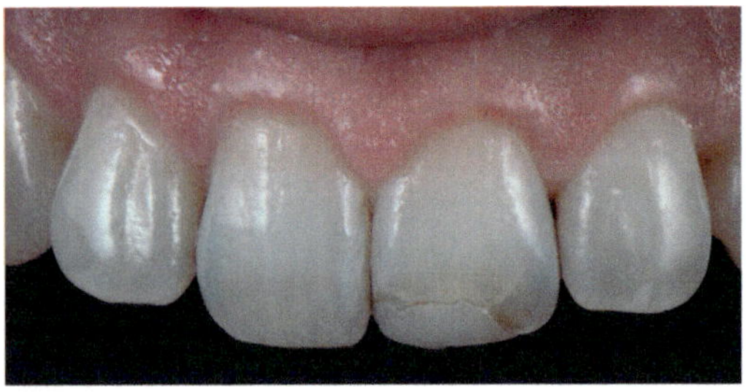

Fig. 7.13 Clinical case of multi-layer build-up technique—modern three-layers: initial situation. (*Photography courtesy of Dr. André Reis*)

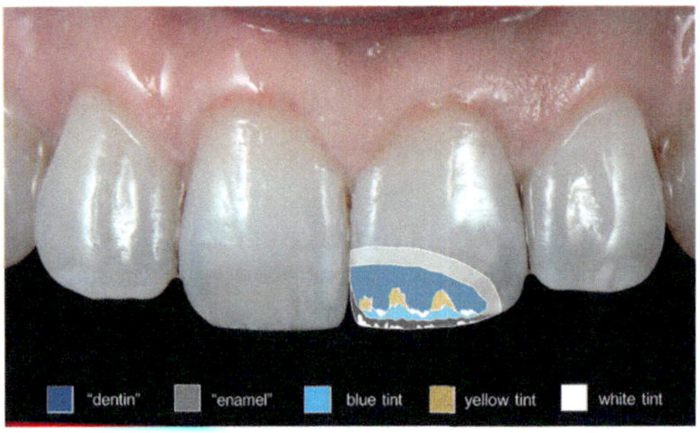

Fig. 7.14 Clinical case of multi-layer build-up technique—modern three-layers: color stratification planning. (*Photography courtesy of Dr. André Reis*)

dentin and enamel layers, that can intensify high-translucent, and opalescent effects, e.g., blue or yellow tint composites use (Figs. 7.13, 7.14 and 7.15), making individual characterization to improve the esthetic [8].

7.1.3.3 Four or More Layers

It comprises a set of four or more different opaque/translucent masses. First, the use of high-opacity materials, named as "dentin" shades, fol-

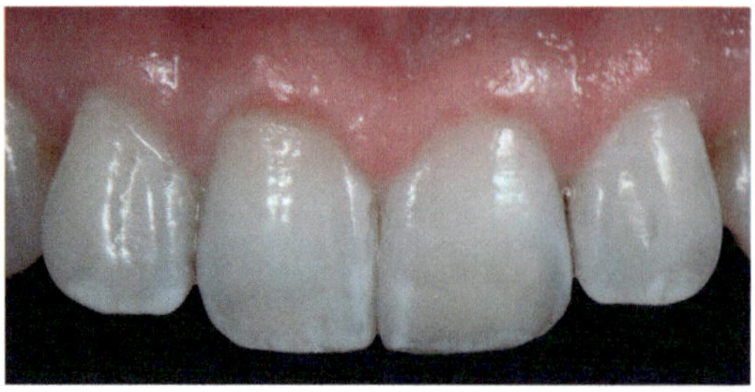

Fig. 7.15 Clinical case of multi-layer build-up technique—modern three-layers: final situation. (*Photography courtesy of Dr. André Reis*)

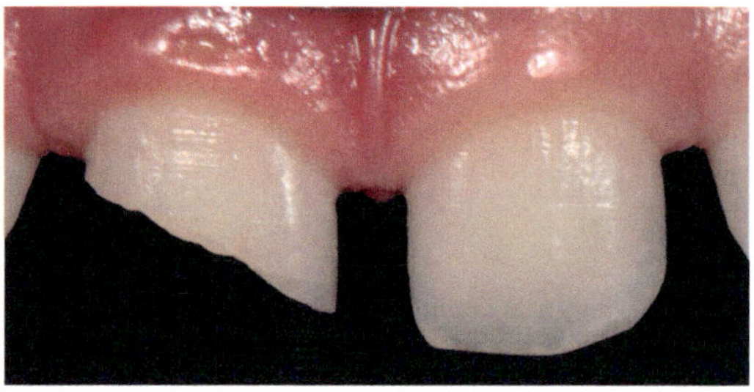

Fig. 7.16 Clinical case of multi-layer build-up technique—*Four or more*-layers: initial situation. (*Photography courtesy of Dr. Monique Solon and Dr. Thais Soares*)

lowed by intermediary opacity, named as "body" shades, then by low-opacity materials, named as "enamel" shades and then by high-translucent materials, named as "translucent," "incisal," or "transparent" shades. Like the classical three-layering, it implies a polychromatic build-up, with opacity and chroma variations from the inside to the outside of restoration. In this technique, the body shades are inserted to stratify the opacity levels between layers in tooth body regions, facilitating camouflage of transition zone between the tooth and the restorative material (Figs. 7.16, 7.17 and 7.18).

7.2 Restorative Planning Using Schematic Drawings

It is a fact that the ability to replace the original morphology of the lost tooth structure is essential to reestablish function, health, and esthetics. However, an optimal understanding of the tooth

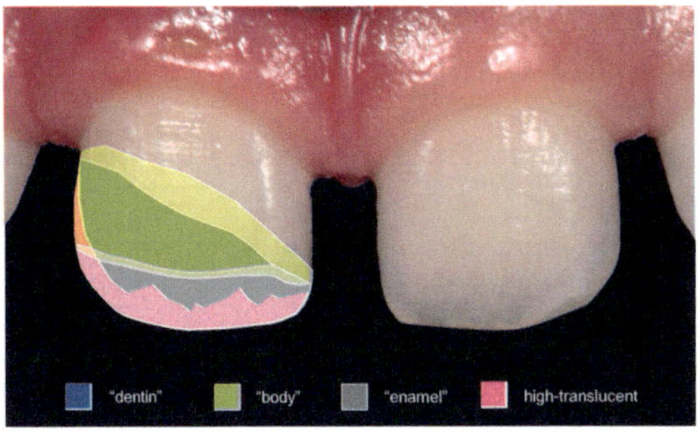

Fig. 7.17 Clinical case of multi-layer build-up technique—*Four or more*-layers: color stratification planning. (*Photography courtesy of Dr. Monique Solon and Dr. Thais Soares*)

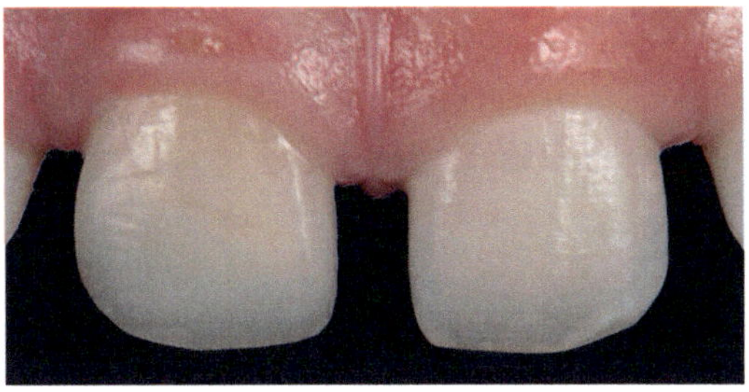

Fig. 7.18 Clinical case of multi-layer build-up technique—*Four or more*-layers: final situation. (*Photography courtesy of Dr. Monique Solon and Dr. Thais Soares*)

morphology can help visualize and better plan the restorative procedure. Schematic drawings have been highly used and recommended for crown fabrication. Most laboratory prescriptions already come with a shade instructions section, including schematic drawings to be chosen or drawn to improve the communication between dentists and laboratories and facilitate color matching.

In direct restorative dentistry, schematic drawing can also facilitate the color match. In order to perfectly achieve biomimetics of the natural tooth, not only the correct shades need to be chosen, but each shade needs to be placed correctly and perfectly mimicking the contralateral tooth (Fig. 7.19a). If correct shades are chosen but incorrectly placed, perfect color matching does not occur (Fig. 7.19b).

As previously described, all conventional composite manufacturers offer dentin and enamel shades. However, body, translucent (or incisal), and effect shades are also available from a few manufacturers, such as Tokuyama (Estelite Omega), 3M (Filtek Supreme Ultra), and Miris 2 (Coltene) (Fig. 7.20a–c). All these different composites have different optical properties to help mimic any natural tooth structure particularities.

7.2.1 One-Layer Build-Up Technique

As previously described in this chapter, the one-layer build-up technique consists of applying just one shade in all extensions of the restoration. This technique is highly effective in small restorations or places where esthetics are not really demanded.

Of course, for this specific technique, schematic drawings are not necessary. However, still, color matching can be challenging. Although the most indicated shade for this technique are body shades [4], esthetic regions where only enamel was lost, enamel shades are usually a better fit.

Specifically for this technique, some manufacturers started fabricating what is now called universal composites. The universal composites consist of a resin-based restorative material for the single-shade technique. These composites come in a universal opacity similar to the body shades (Fig. 7.21).

Some books and authors also call this technique the *Chameleon technique* due to the monochromatic build-up of the restoration with a single shaded material [4]. However, the Chameleon effect is known as the phenomena of perfectly blending with the surrounding background. However, of course, such situation only happens when color matching is perfect. For this reason, some manufacturers are now fabricating and claiming some composites have a true chameleon effect. These composites are a single uncolored shade able to blend with the surrounding tooth structure perfectly. The manufacturers claim the target refraction of light creates structural color in the yellow–red range and reflect the surrounding real tooth color. Examples of chameleon effect composites are

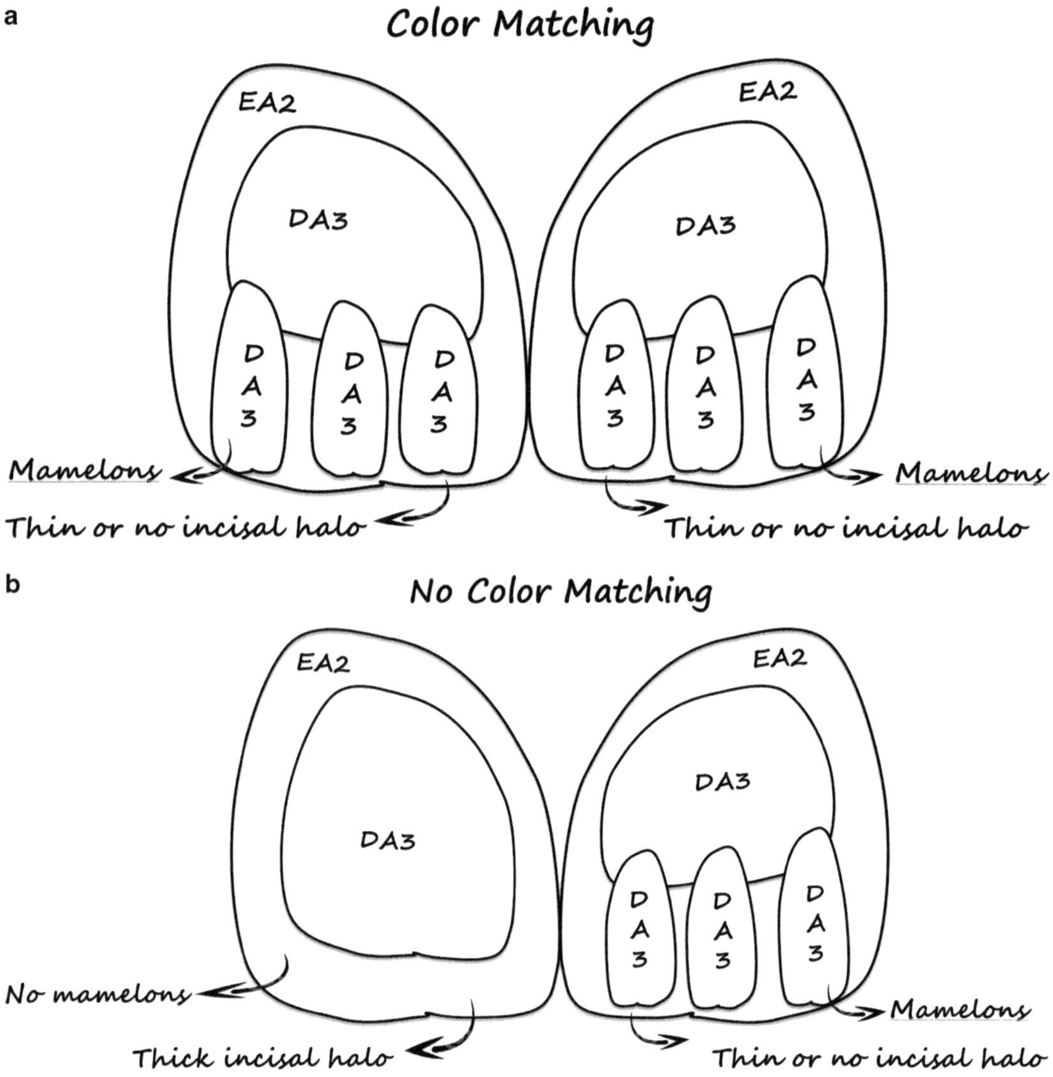

Fig. 7.19 Example of correct shade selection with: (**a**) correct layering placement and (**b**) incorrect layering placement, and color matching

the Omnichroma (Tokuyama) (Fig. 7.22a). The Omnichroma composite also offer a blocker shade to be used over dark discolored tooth structures and facilitating correct color matching (Fig. 7.22b).

The literature shows these composites cannot perfectly blend with the surrounding tooth structure as the multi-layer build-up technique. However, they do have a high clinical color matching acceptance [9–12]. It is worthwhile to mention that these composites are also helpful in simplifying color selection and minimizing clinical errors when the one-layer build-up technique is indicated.

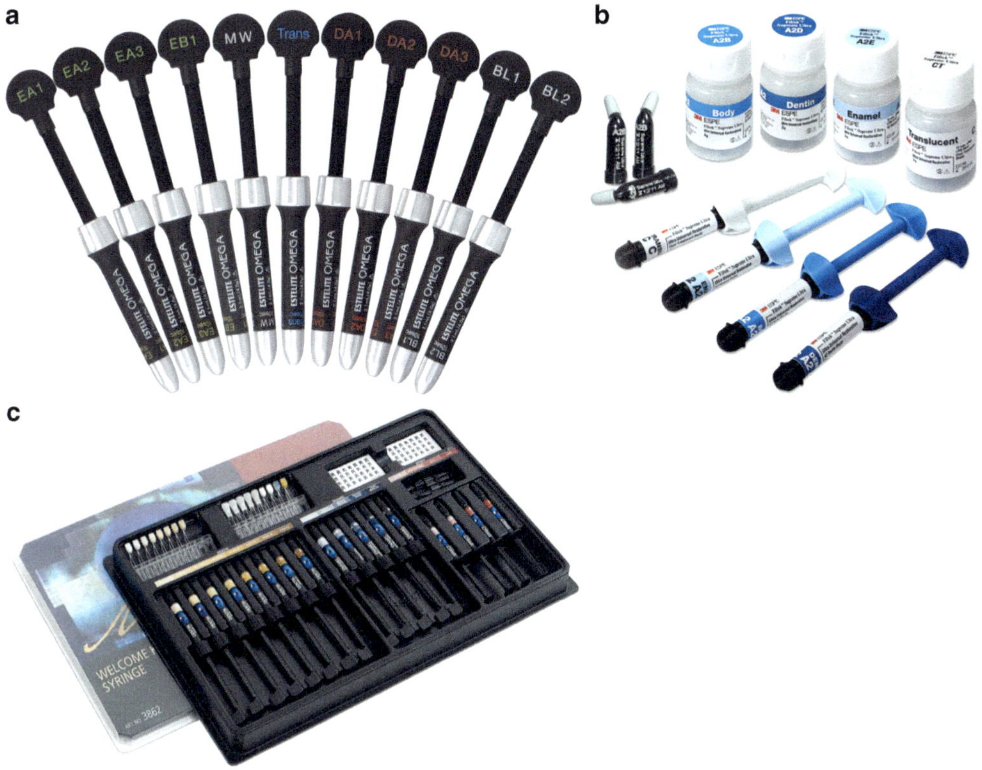

Fig. 7.20 Conventional composites: (**a**) Estelite Omega (Tokuyama); (**b**) Filtek Supreme Ultra (3M); and Miris 2 (Coltene). (*Photography courtesy of Tokuyama Dental, 3M and Coltene*)

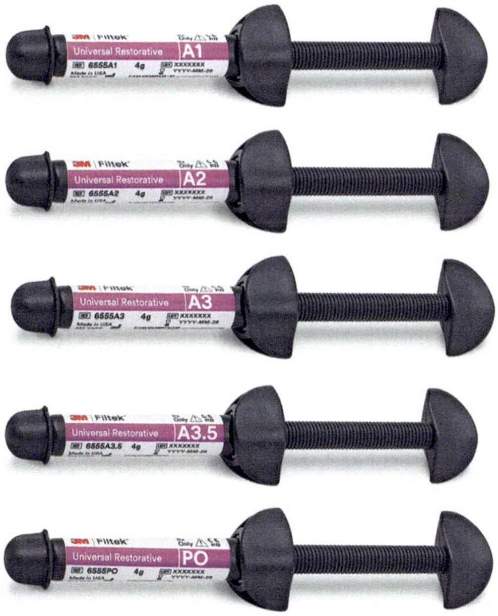

Fig. 7.21 Filtek universal composites (3M). (*Photography courtesy of 3M*)

7.2.2 Two-Layers Build-Up Technique

The two-layers build-up technique is sub-classified into two categories: the *Classical two-layering* and the *Natural two-layering*. The main difference between these two categories is the type of opaque and translucent composites combined to mimic dentin and enamel. Regardless of the terminology, what will dictate what composite will be used is the one that better mimics the color and the translucency properties of the natural tooth being reconstructed. For this, a quick mock-up with the two shades layered can help to identify the more appropriate combinations (Fig. 7.23a) before the final restorative procedure (Fig. 7.23b).

As illustrated in Fig. 7.24a–f, the schematic drawings for the two-layer build-up technique is focused on where the dentin or body will be placed and shaped following the morphology of the natural dentin and its characteristics.

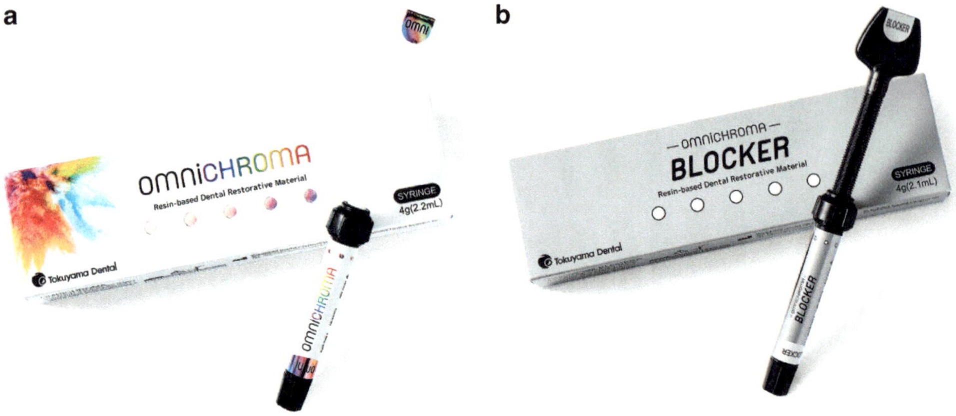

Fig. 7.22 Chameleon effect composite: (**a**) Omnichroma (Tokuyama) and its (**b**) blocker. (*Photography courtesy of Tokuyama Dental*)

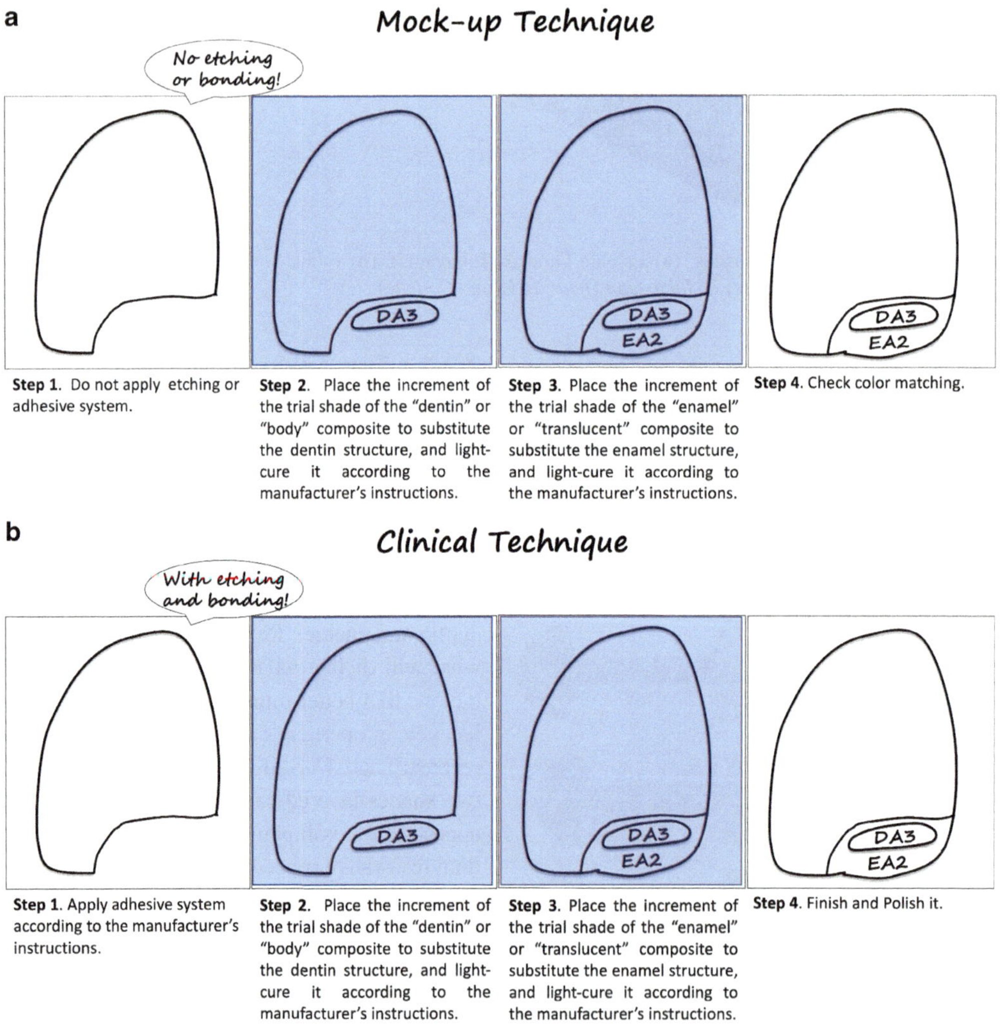

Fig. 7.23 (**a**) Mock-up technique prior. (**b**) Final restorative technique

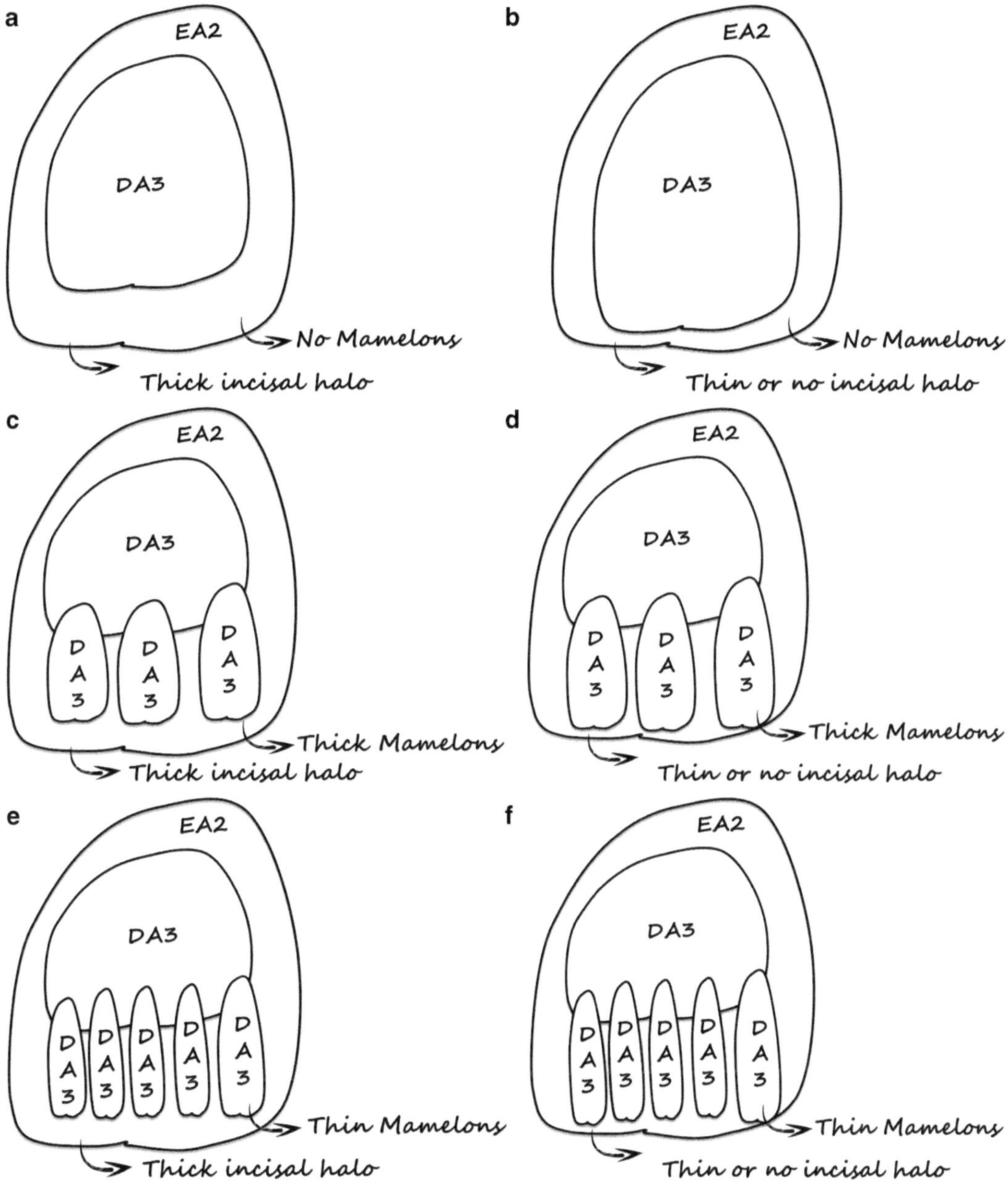

Fig. 7.24 (**a**–**f**) Schematic drawings of two-layers build-up technique examples

7.2.3 Multi-Layers Build-Up Technique

7.2.3.1 Classical Three Layers

This technique comprises the use of three different opacity masses: dentin, enamel, and translucent, or also called incisal or transparent depending on the manufacturer. For this technique, the schematic drawing is focused on where the dentin, enamel, and translucent shades will be placed, as well as how the dentin is shaped following the morphology of the natural dentin and its characteristics (Fig. 7.25).

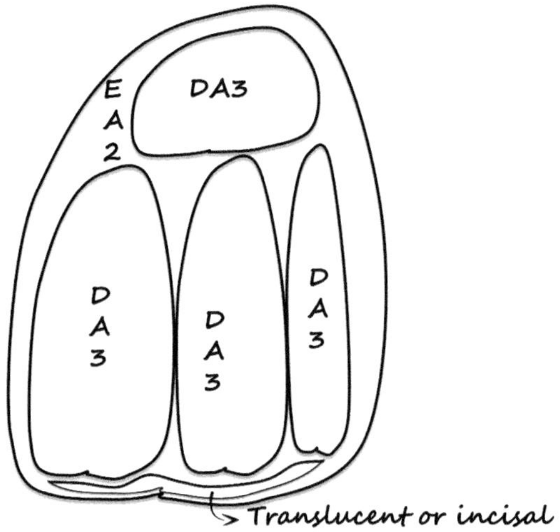

Fig. 7.25 Schematic drawing of classical three-layering technique example

7.2.3.2 Modern Three Layers

The main difference between this technique and the two-layers build-up is the addition of "effect" materials between dentin/body and enamel/translucent layers to reproduce anatomic details for individual characterization.

For this technique, the schematic drawing not only focuses on where the dentin or body will be placed and shaped but where the effect material will be placed and shaped following the anatomical defect or characteristic that is being reproduced (Fig. 7.26a–c).

7.2.3.3 Four or More-Layers

This technique comprises the use of four or more different opacity masses: dentin, body, enamel, and translucent. For this technique, the schematic

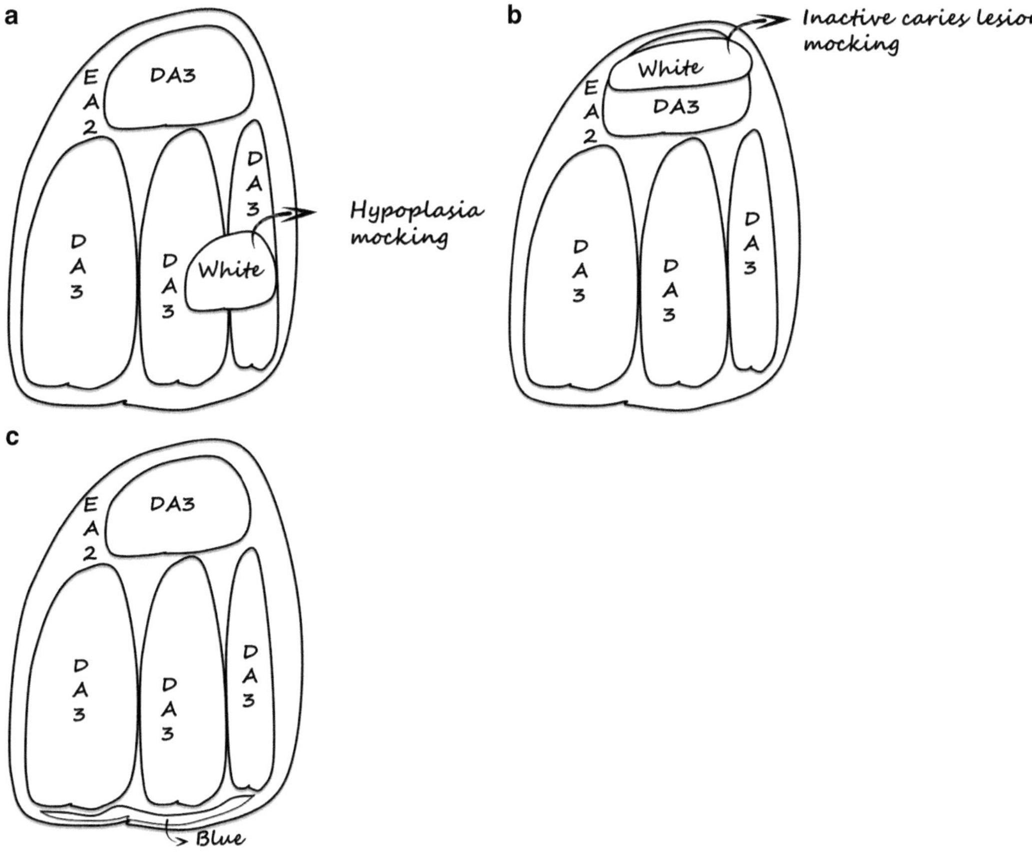

Fig. 7.26 Schematic drawings of modern three-layering technique examples: (**a**) using white effect to mock a hypoplasia defect; (**b**) using white effect to mock an inactive carious lesion on the neck following the contour of the gum line; (**c**) using blue effect to mock opalescence of incisal halo

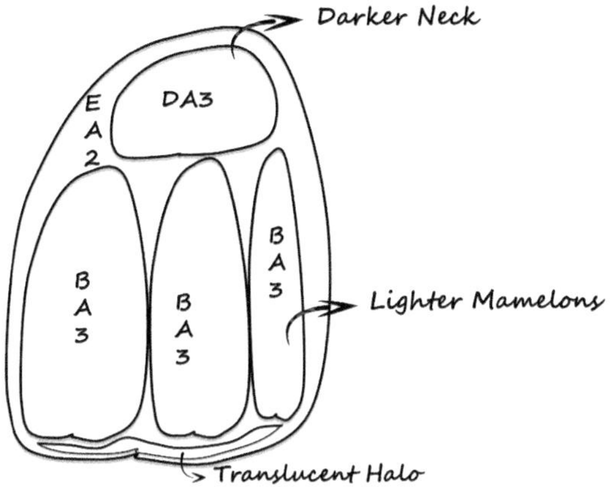

Fig. 7.27 Schematic drawing of classical four or more-layers technique

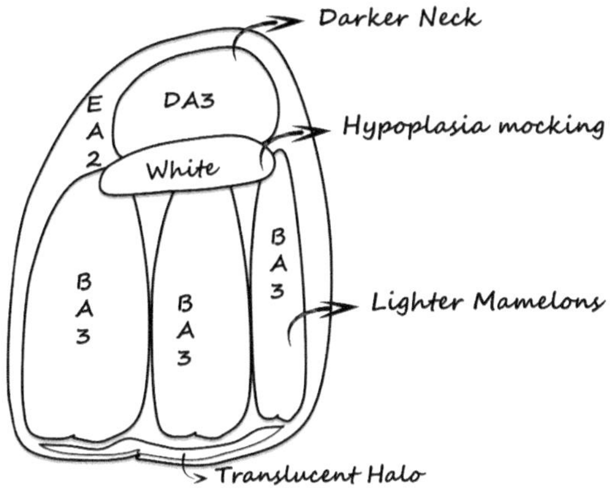

Fig. 7.28 Schematic drawing of classical four or more-layers technique including "effect" material

drawing is focused on where the dentin, body, enamel, and translucent shades will be placed, as well as how the dentin is shaped following the morphology of the natural dentin and its characteristics (Fig. 7.27).

It is important to point out that "effect" materials can also be applied in this technique. In these cases, the schematic drawing should also include where the effect material will be placed and how it will be shaped following the anatomical defect or characteristic that is being reproduced (Fig. 7.28).

References

1. Dietschi D, Fahl N Jr. Shading concepts and layering techniques to master direct anterior composite restorations: an update. Br Dent J. 2016;221(12):765–71.
2. Dietschi D. Layering concepts in anterior composite restorations. J Adhes Dent. 2001;3(1):71–80.
3. Bayindir F, Gozalo-Diaz D, Kim-Pusateri S, Wee AG. Incisal translucency of vital natural unrestored teeth: a clinical study. J Esthet Restor Dent. 2012;24(5):335–43.
4. Fahl N Jr. Single-shaded direct anterior composite restorations: a simplified technique for enhanced results. Compend Contin Educ Dent. 2012;33(2):150–4.
5. Dietschi D. Free-hand bonding in the esthetic treatment of anterior teeth: creating the illusion. J Esthet Dent. 1997;9(4):156–64.
6. Ardu S, Krejci I. Biomimetic direct composite stratification technique for the restoration of anterior teeth. (Erratum in: Quintessence Int. 2006 May;37(5):408). Quintessence Int. 2006;37(3):167–74.
7. Dietschi D, Ardu S, Krejci I. A new shading concept based on natural tooth color applied to direct composite restorations. Quintessence Int. 2006;37(2):91–102.
8. Fahl N Jr. Achieving ultimate anterior esthetics with a new microhybrid composite. Compend Contin Educ Dent Suppl. 2000;26:4–13.
9. Abreu JLB, Sampaio CS, Jalkh EBB, Hirata R. Analysis of the color matching of universal resin composites in anterior teeth. J Esthet Restor Dent. 2021;33(2):269–76.
10. Iyer RS, Babani VR, Yaman P, Dennison J. Color matching using instrumental and visual methods for single, group, and multi-shade composite resins. J Esthet Restor Dent. 2021;33(2):394–400.
11. Sanchez NP, Powers JM, Paravina RD. Instrumental and visual evaluation of the color adjustment potention of resin composites. J Esthet Rest Dent. 2019;31(5):465–70.
12. Optical behavior of one-shaded resin-based composites. Dent Mater. 2021;37(5):840–8.

Finishing and Polishing

8

Alex J. Delgado

8.1 Finishing and Polishing Importance

Finishing and polishing composite restorations is an essential procedure for the longevity of the restoration and the tooth [1, 2]. A well-contoured, finished, and polished restoration will promote oral health, serve functionality, and preserve esthetics. Finishing is the gross reduction of the restorative material to obtain an anatomical contour of the restoration and make the margins undetectable, while polishing makes the surface smooth and lustrous [3, 4] (Figs. 8.1 and 8.2). Finishing and polishing goals are to obtain the desired anatomy, proper occlusion, and functionality, reduce roughness, and increase surface smoothness to recreate nature.

Appropriate instrumentation must be selected according to the specific surface being contoured [5]. Lack of proper finishing and polishing procedures can compromise marginal integrity, leading to staining and discoloration of the restoration, gingival inflammation or irritation, and plaque accumulation that could result in recurrent caries (Fig. 8.3) [1].

Instrumentation for finishing and polishing available to the clinicians include (1) fluted carbide burs, (2) diamond burs, (3) coated aluminum oxide disc, (4) rubber impregnated rubber cups, points, and discs, (5) interproximal strips, (6) polishing brushes, wheels, and felts, and (7) polishing pastes. The most studied and common instruments for contouring a restoration are the fluted carbides, diamond burs, coated aluminum discs, and impregnated rubber cups, points, and discs. These finishing and polishing instruments are often offered in different degrees of abrasiveness, come in sets, and should be used in the proper sequence, working gradually from the course to the finest [1, 2]. The clinician must also take into general consideration factors such as the type of handpiece (friction grip or latch), the rotation per minute recommended by the manufacture, and the pressure applied to each of these instruments. Also, local considerations must be considered, for instance, the grit of abrasiveness, the number of blades, if the instrument is disposable or if it should be in a dry or wet condition [6, 7]. It is also worth mentioning that it is crucial to know the effect of polishing direction on the marginal adaptation of the restoration. A study demonstrated a significant difference in the marginal adaptation when polishing is accomplished from resin-based composites to tooth structure instead of tooth to resin [8].

Obtaining an anatomical contoured of the restoration will provide better oral health preventing gingival inflammation and plaque accumulation because the proper anatomy will help the spillway,

A. J. Delgado (✉)
Department of Restorative Dental Sciences, College of Dentistry, University of Florida, Gainesville, FL, USA
e-mail: ADelgado@dental.ufl.edu

D. Oliveira (ed.), *Color Science and Shade Selection in Operative Dentistry*,
https://doi.org/10.1007/978-3-030-99173-9_8

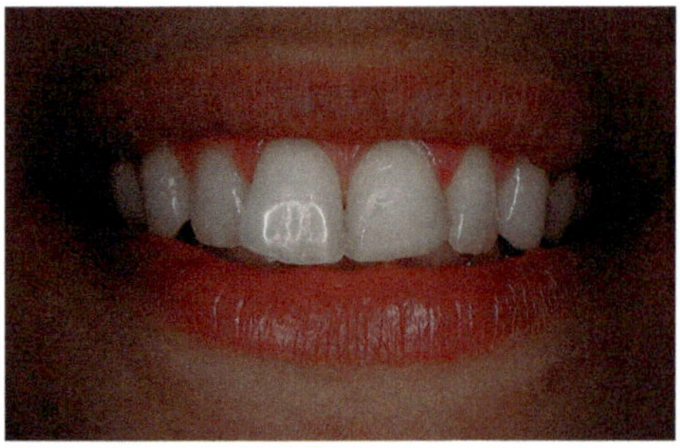

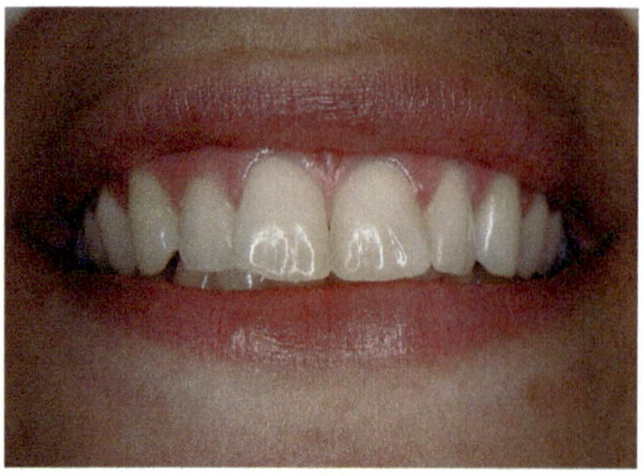

Figs. 8.1 and 8.2 Clinical case before and after finishing and polishing of the composite restoration. (*Photography courtesy of Dr. Dayane Oliveira* et al.)

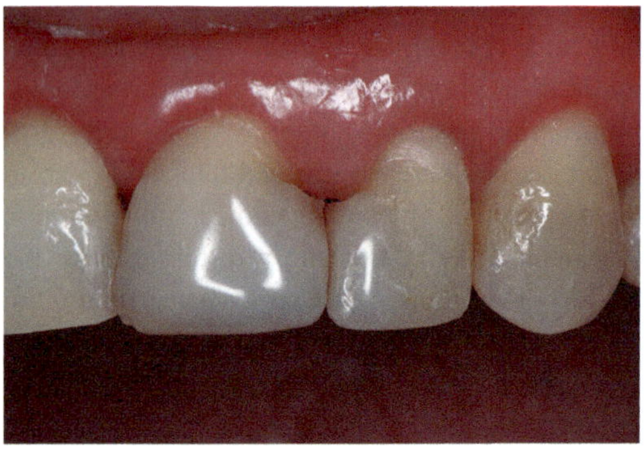

Fig. 8.3 Discoloration and gingival inflammation due to marginal discrepancy of the composite restoration. (*Photography courtesy of Dr. Vinicius Salgado*)

which are grooves, embrasures, or channels through which food particles may pass from occlusal surfaces of the teeth during the masticatory process and adds in the self-cleansing process [9].

Staining and discoloring the restoration might be a consequence of the lack of fine finishing, which is the process to remove scratches and improve the surface smoothness sufficiently enough to polish. Finishing and polishing procedures can be detrimental to the surface of restoration and, more importantly, to the marginal integrity. Marginal integrity defects can lead to microleaking in the enamel and dentin interface [10]. The marginal gap can accumulate external staining from extrinsic sources and result in marginal leaking, recurrent caries, and affecting the pulp tissue [11]. Therefore, it is important for the tooth vitality and the longevity of the restoration that possible marginal gaps are prevented. Finishing and polishing techniques are under the clinician's control and are essential to achieve good marginal integrity.

No minimum marginal gap has been identified as acceptable for composite restorations. The literature is controversial in this regard. A study reported that a gap of less than 1 μm is required to prevent bacterial infiltration. However, some toxins can still harm the tooth [11–13].

Over the past decades, the importance of esthetics dentistry has become more evident. In current clinical treatment, many types of restorations are available for the replacement of lost tooth structure. The introduction of composite restorations introduced a new concept in esthetic dentistry and the development of many types of resin-based composites and techniques that can completely mimic the different characteristics of the natural tooth (see further details in Chaps. 2 and 7).

8.2 Finishing and Polishing Concept

Finishing and polishing can be divided into four steps: Gross finishing, Contouring, Fine finishing, and Polishing (Fig. 8.4).

Gross finishing is the removal of the resin-based composite gross excess to create a close shape to the tooth's contour. This step is typically accomplished by using coarse grits instruments (green and blue stripe).

Contouring is the step that involves establishing the outline and functional form of the restoration. In this step, the margin integrity should be

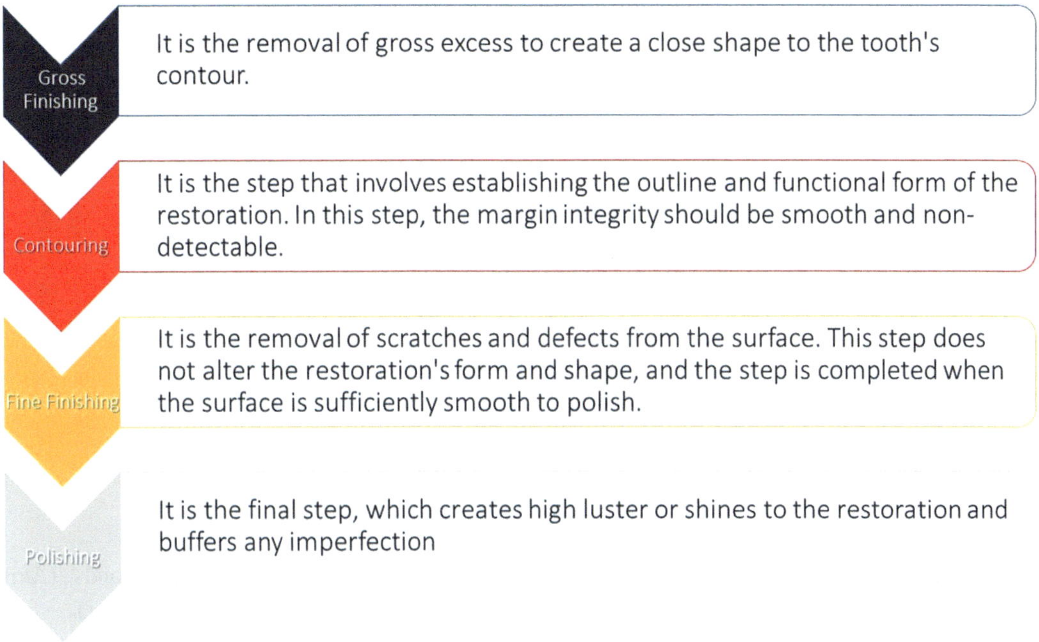

Fig. 8.4 Steps for finishing and polishing resin-based composite restorations

smooth and non-detectable. This step is usually accomplished with fine grist (red strips).

Fine finishing is the removal of scratches and defects from the surface. This step does not alter the restoration's form and shape, and the step is completed when the surface is sufficiently smooth to polish. This step is merely complete with superfine instrumentation (yellow strips).

Polishing is the final step, which creates high luster or shines to the restoration and buffers any imperfection. For this step, the instrumentation should be ultrafine (white strips).

8.3 Finishing and Polishing Systems

8.3.1 Fluted Carbide Finishing Burs

Fluted carbide finishing burs are made of tungsten carbide, a more rigid metal than steel, and can withstand high temperatures. The fact that these burs are made of such rigid and resistant metal, they can maintain a sharp cutting edge, keeping the cutting efficiency after many uses without becoming dull very easily. However, carbides burs under high pressure can become brittle and therefore fracture. Fluted carbide burs come with 8, 12, 15, 16, 20, 30, and 40 flutes (Fig. 8.5).

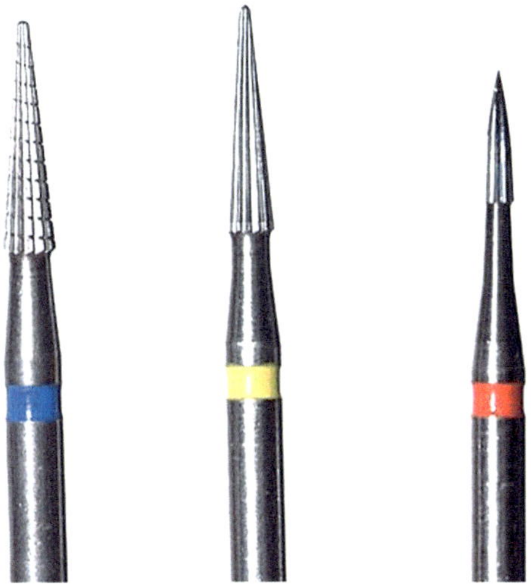

Fig. 8.5 Fluted carbides burs. Red (8 μm), blue (12 μm), yellow (30 μm), and white (40 μm). (*Photography courtesy of Dr. Fernando Haddock*)

These burs can be used for any direct restorative material. The greater the flutes, the less aggressive the instrument is. For contouring, the 8 and 12 fluted burs are typically used, but their use does not result in a well-polished surface. The use of 15–30 fluted burs will result in fine finishing, leaving the surface ready for the polishing step. 40 fluted is the final step and will polish the restoration without altering the final surface. Fluted carbide burs have various shapes available, and each shape is designed for a specific purpose. The most common shapes used during finishing and polishing are the footballs and the flames. Two commercially available fluted burs in the market are the ET series (Brasseler USA) and the SE series (SS White).

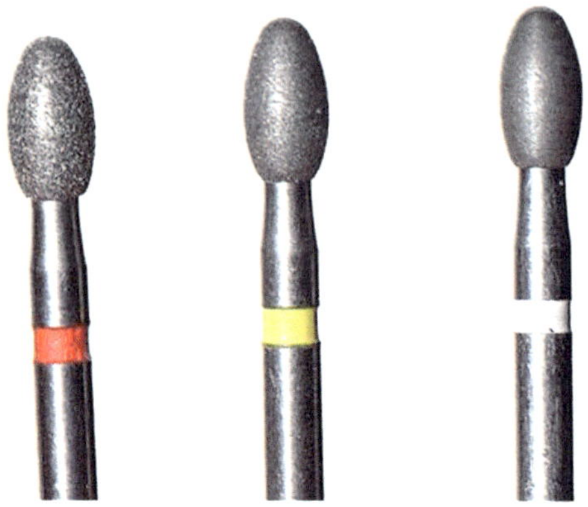

Fig. 8.6 Diamonds burs showing the difference in the grits from coarse to superfine. (*Photography courtesy of Dr. Fernando Haddock*)

8.3.2 Diamond Finishing Burs

Diamond burs consist of a metal-based blank surface coated with powdered diamond abrasive particles bonded by a metallic adhesive. Diamond is the harder cutting material in Dentistry, and it is superior in its cutting efficiency over other finishing and polishing instruments. Unlike fluted carbide burs, diamonds rely on the grinding by abrasiveness particles rather than blades cutting action. Diamonds' particles can vary in size and shape. Thus, allowing finishing and polishing results in a shorter period. However, their life span is shorter than fluted carbide burs. The diamond particles eventually are flaked off from the metal-based blank surface due to the friction over time. Coarse diamond burs have a range of 50–150 μm, while medium grits are usually 40 μm, fine grits are 25–30 μm, the extra-fine are usually 12–15 μm, and superfine 7–8 μm (Fig. 8.6). The clinical performance of diamond burs depends on the size and shape distribution of the diamond particles, but its hardness is sufficient for polishing direct and indirect materials [3, 14–16]. The manufactures recommend using gentle wiping strokes with these instruments and with water irrigation, preferably, to avoid heat. Some of the most common diamond burs commercially available in the market are the ET Series (Brasseler), the NTI Diamonds (Axis Dental), and the Solo Diamond (Premier).

8.3.2.1 Fluted Carbide Finishing Burs vs. Diamond Finishing Burs

The clinician must understand the difference between both instruments. Fluted carbides burs remove restorative material by slicing or shaving away the composite while diamond burs grind away the material. In the end, both instruments can achieve a smooth surface.

8.3.2.2 Finishing Burs Shapes and Their Applications

There are several bur shapes accordingly to different applications. The most used ones are the taper finishing, the flame, and the football. The taper finishing is mainly indicated for flat surfaces, including facial and margin areas. The flame is mainly indicated for occlusal areas. The football is mainly indicated for occlusal (pointed football) and cingulum areas (round football).

8.3.3 Impregnated Aluminum Oxide Discs

Impregnated aluminum oxide discs are fabricated by securing abrasive particles of a chemical compound of aluminum and oxygen to a flexible

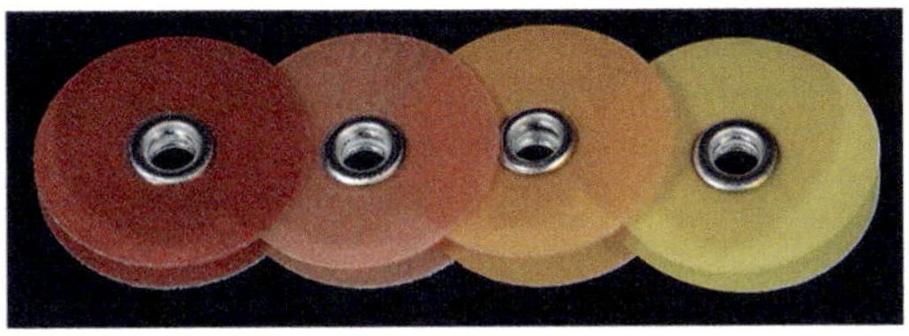

Fig. 8.7 Sof-Lex discs (3MESPE) and Super Snap (Shofu)

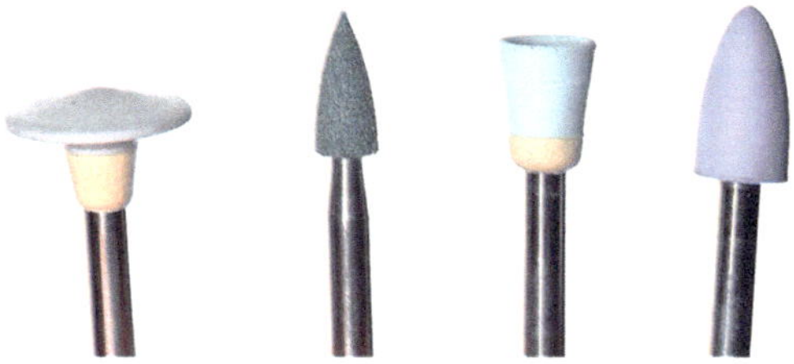

Fig. 8.8 Cups, discs, and flames silicon impregnated rubber. (*Photography courtesy of Dr. Fernando Haddock*)

backing material that could be paper or mylar (Fig. 8.7). These particles are retained on the disc by a polymeric adhesive coating layer. Aluminum oxide can be used to finish and polish composites, ceramics, and even enamel [2]. The most common examples of impregnated aluminum oxide discs commercially available in the market include the Sof-Lex discs (3M ESPE, St Paul, MN) and the Super Snap discs (Shofu Dental Corp, Menlo Park, CA). Both discs have a coarse disc with about 80–100 μm, a medium of around 40 μm, fine with 24 μm, and superfine with 8 μm. One advantage of the discs is that they are positioned in a mandrel, making it easier to exchange the discs when needed. The Sof-Lex has the advantage of being flipped to address different surface areas. Still, a significant drawback is that they will flatten surfaces if not positioned with caution and cannot be used in concave areas. Their main applications are for use in proximal and facial surfaces.

8.3.4 Impregnated Rubber Cups, Points, and Discs

These instruments come in different shapes, such as cups, points, and discs. They are made of rubber or elastomeric materials with bonded abrasive coatings such as aluminum oxide, silicon dioxide or silicon carbide, zirconium oxide, or diamond particles. The most popular abrasive coating is aluminum oxide. These instruments can be used in all types of composites and ceramics. These instruments possess a low cutting efficiency but can be used for contouring. The cups, discs, and points come in latch-type and should be used under 10,000 RPM with water irrigation (Fig. 8.8). These instruments come with different grits ranging from 40 to 6 μm for polishing [14, 15]. The main indications for discs are for use in proximal and facial surfaces, while points are for use in occlusal and cingulum surfaces, and cups are for use in cusp tips are and overall flat surfaces.

A few companies have developed a one-step polisher, such as the PoGo (Dentsply Sirona), the OneGloss, (Shofu INC), or the OptraPol (Ivoclar). These are single-use, diamond-impregnated, or aluminum oxide polishers for the final polishing of composites, and they are available in cups, flames, and discs shapes.

8.3.5 Interproximal Strips

Interproximal strips are flexible strips made of mylar (polyester) or metal with an aluminum oxide particles coating. Finishing strips are made for the interproximal areas and facilitate the finishing of any margin discrepancies or roughness to avoid plaque accumulation in the proximal surfaces. Finishing strips are suitable for flat and convex surfaces. These strips come in two different sizes, regular and narrow, to give the dentist flexibility to be working in the interproximal areas in different clinical scenarios. The narrow strips are excellent to avoid removing or opening the proximal contact and protect the soft tissue from damage while using the strips near the gums. If the contact is broad or too tight, these strips are ideal for lightening the contact. Usually, the regular can be used in patients with bone loss or gingival recession. The strips should be curved over the restoration in an "S" motion (Fig. 8.9) to ensure correct contour. These strips come in dif-

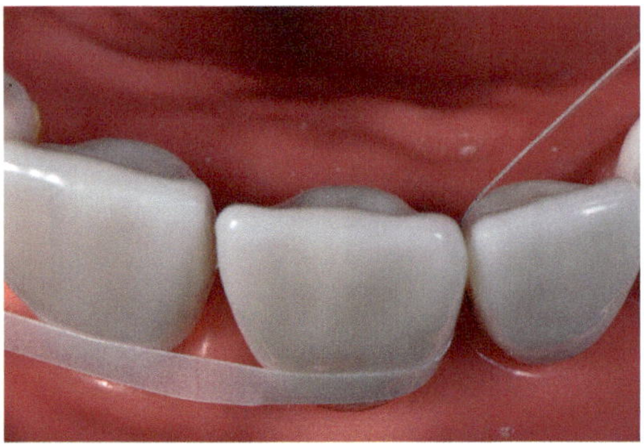

Fig. 8.9 Polishing strips. (*Photography courtesy of Dr. Dayane Oliveira and Dr. Mateus Garcia Rocha*)

ferent grits of abrasiveness from medium to fine and intend to remove resin material excesses. Before using these strips, the interproximal area should be assessed visually and tactile with the explorer, and thin and unwaxed floss should be passed between the contacts to ensure that the floss does not fray or catch. These strips have a center part where no abrasive is present to facilitate passing through the contact area and reaching the proximal surfaces without removing or opening the proximal contact. The metal strips are far more aggressive than the polyester strips, and they come with coarse to superfine grits, and they also have serrated strips to open contacts. More caution should be used with these products. Examples of polishing strips commercially available in the market are the Sof-Lex (3MESPE), the FlexiDiamonds Finishing Strips (Cosmodent), the EPITEX (GC America), and the NTI Diamond (Kerr) [16]

8.3.6 Impregnated Polishing Brushes

The brushes intend to reach deep grooves, fissures, and depressions without removing the restoration's anatomy. These brushes have bristles impregnated with various abrasiveness particles, as mentioned previously in this chapter. The brushes come in two different sizes, small, and large, and in two different shapes, cups, and flames (Fig. 8.10). These brushes are indicated for composites, ceramics, and enamel. The manufacturer recommends using the brush at a maximum speed of 3000 rpm and intermittent or dabbing brush movements. Water irrigation can be used, but it is not mandatory. Some examples of impregnated brushes commercially available in the market are the Jiffy (Ultradent), Groovy Diamond Polishing Brush (Clinician Choice), and the Jazz Polishers (SS White Dental Inc) [16].

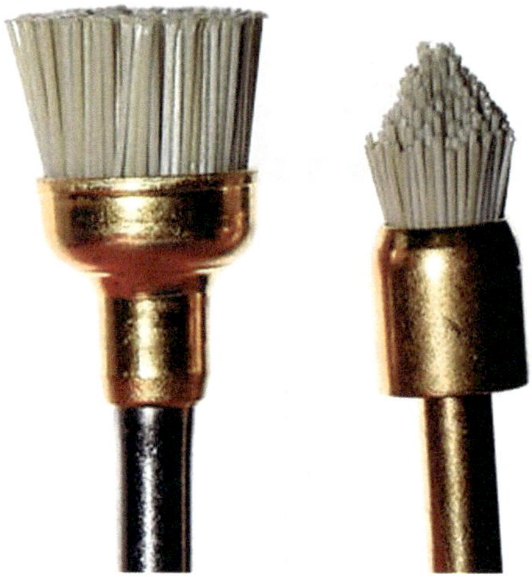

Fig. 8.10 Impregnated brushes: flame and cup shapes. (*Photography courtesy of Dr. Fernando Haddock*)

8.3.7 Impregnated Wheels

Polishing wheels are pre-mounted on mandrels and come impregnated with diamond particles. They are very popular in the market and come in different abrasiveness. Lately, a new type of wheel has come out in the market, and those are the flexible wheels, which are rubber fingers with embedded particles throughout the wheel, making it very efficient and easy to use (Fig. 8.11). Examples of flexible wheels commercially available in the market are the Sof-Lex Spiral Wheels (3M ESPE) and the BioShine (Brasseler USA) [15].

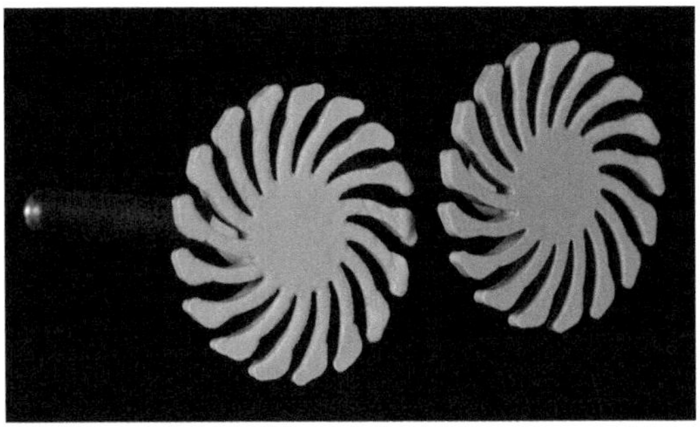

Fig. 8.11 Impregnated wheels. (*Photography courtesy of Dr. Dayane Oliveira and Dr. Mateus Garcia Rocha*)

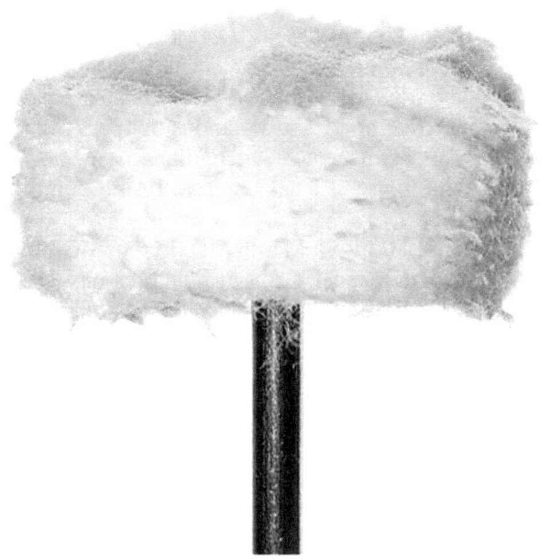

Fig. 8.12 Polishing wheel felt and polishing pastes. (*Photography courtesy of Dr. Fernando Haddock*)

8.3.8 Felts and Polishing Pastes

The felts are made of fine white wool, and they are designed to be used in combination with polishing pates to buffer polishing imperfection (Fig. 8.12). Polishing pastes are typically glycerin-based with suspended diamond particles or ultrafine aluminum oxide particles. The particle sizes are usually not greater than 6–7 μm, and the majority are less than 1 μm. These pastes should be used with water irrigation to avoid the crystallization of the silica. The crystals could scratch the surface, resulting in a rougher surface [17, 18].

8.3.9 Liquid Polishing Systems

Liquid polishing systems are also commercially available in the market. This system is a low viscous light-cured resin that contains high molecular weight monomers diluted in a solvent. Thus, this low viscous liquid is capable of infiltrating the surface porosities of the restoration. This way, after photo-activation, the restoration has a smoother and glossy surface. Although these liquid polishing systems have an easy and low-time consuming technique and excellent initial smooth and gloss results, they have low wear resistance that leads to lower gloss retention compared to the other polishing systems over time. Thus, for esthetics, the most important is not only to choose an adequate type of resin composite according to esthetical and functional needs but also to perform adequate finishing and polishing techniques.

8.4 The Artistic Element in Finishing and Polishing

8.4.1 Illusion Effects

Composite restorations have achieved an important milestone in Esthetic Dentistry, but there is an area where nature can be brought closer. Sometimes, the clinicians can incorporate texture or simply modify the symmetry or proportionality of the final restoration. Creating illusions of length is an artistic element that can be incorporated and made by different instruments already mentioned above. A tooth may look longer if the gingival height of contour is moved closer to the gingival margin or shorter if the same is moved more incisally. An illusion of the width can be created by moving the mesial and distal line angles closer (narrowing) or apart (widening).

Surface texture will make the restoration more natural because natural teeth are not entirely flat or free of defects. They possess concavities, convexity, scratches, and areas of stippling. Different tooth structures have different optical properties.

That is why it is crucial to understand how the light is reflected by different types of composites. Still, the light reflection is different when you have texture on the surface, and it is essential to assess the light reflection and propagation after the final polishing. Adding texture to the restoration may improve this phenomenon.

8.4.2 Surface Texture

Younger teeth have significant characterization, while older patients have less anatomy and texture because of the gradually physiological wear. In younger patients, teeth carry wavelike grooves in the cervical and mid area from the mesial line angle to the distal line angle called perikymata. These stripes never cross each other, and they are circumferential, and they will create a great deal on the reflection of the light [19].

References

1. Jefferies SR. The art and science of abrasive finishing and polishing in restorative dentistry. Dent Clin N Am. 1998;42(4):613–27.
2. Jefferies SR. Abrasive finishing and polishing in restorative dentistry: a state-of-the-art review. Dent Clin N Am. 2007;51(2):379–97.
3. Anunsavice K, Shen C, Rawls HR. Phillips' science of dental materials. 12th ed. Amsterdam: Elsevier; 2012.
4. Oliveira DCRS, Oliveira LV, Castro NA, Paulillo LAMS, Pereira GDS. Esthetic results using composite resin restorations: nature-like results. Clin Inte J Braz Dent. 2011;7(2):1780184.
5. Ritter AV, Boushell L, Walter R. Sturdevant's art and science of operative dentistry. Amsterdam: Elsevier; 2018.
6. Delgado AJ, Ritter AV, Donovan TE, Ziemiecki T, Heymann HO. Effect of finishing techniques on the marginal integrity of resin-based composite and resin-modified glass ionomer restoration. J Esthet Restor Dent. 2015;27(4):184–93.
7. Maresca C, Pimenta LA, Heymann HO, Ziemiecki TL, Ritter AV. Effect of finishing instrumentation on the marginal integrity of resin-based composite restorations. J Esthet Restor Dent. 2010;22(2):104–12.
8. St-Pierre L, Bergeron C, Qian F, Hernández MM, Kolker JL, Cobb DS, Vargas MA. Effect of polishing direction on the marginal adaptation of composite resin restorations. J Esthet Restor Dent. 2013;25(2):125–38.
9. Ash MM. Wheeler's dental anatomy, physiology, and occlusion. 10th ed. Amsterdam: Elsevier; 2015.
10. ADA Council on Scientific Affairs. ADA Council on dental benefit programs. J Am Dent Assoc. 1998;129(11):1627–8.
11. Taylor MJ, Lynch E. Marginal adaptation. J Dent. 1993;21(5):265–73.
12. Soncini JA, Maserejian NN, Trachtenberg F, Tavares M, Hayes C. The longevity of amalgam versus compomer/composite restorations in posterior primary and permanent teeth: findings from the New England Children's amalgam trial. J Am Dent Assoc. 2007;138(6):763–72.
13. Bernardo M, Luis H, Martin MD, Leroux BG, Rue T, Leitão J, DeRouen TA. Survival and reasons for failure of amalgam versus composite posterior restorations placed in a randomized clinical trial. J Am Dent Assoc. 2007;138(6):775–83.
14. Watanabe T, Miyazaki M, Takamizawa T, Kurokawa H, Rikuta A, Ando S. Influence of polishing duration on surface roughness of resin composites. J Oral Sci. 2005;47(1):21–5.
15. Türkün LS, Türkün M. The effect of one-step polishing system on the surface roughness of three esthetic resin composite materials. Oper Dent. 2004;29(2):203–11.
16. Powers JM, Sakaguhi RL. Craig's restorative dental materials. 10th ed. St. Louis: Mosby; 1997. p. 231.
17. Whitehead SA, Wilson NH. The nature and effects of composite finishing pastes. J Dent. 1989;17(5):234–40. https://doi.org/10.1016/0300-5712(89)90174-7.
18. Tjan AH, Chan CA. The polishability of posterior composites. J Prosthet Dent. 1989;61(2):138–46.
19. Maia RR, Oliveira D, D'Antonio T, Qian F, Skiff F. Double-layer build-up technique: laser evaluation of light propagation in dental substrates and dental composites. Int J Esthet Dent. 2018;13(4):538–49.

Color Mismatch Between the Restoration and the Natural Tooth Over Time

9

Luis Felipe Jochims Schneider
and Larissa Maria Assad Cavalcante

9.1 Color Change in Resin Composite Restorations

Resin composites represent a significant advance in the field of restorative, conservative, and esthetic dentistry and today are the most-used direct material worldwide [1]. This has not always been the case, however, and early problems associated with the adhesion process, unsatisfactory physicochemical properties, high polymerization shrinkage, and excessive wear have necessitated an evolution in resin composite manufacturing techniques [2]. Miletic [3] reported that the significant advances in resin composite technology encompass modifications in (a) the curing pathway (between the mid-1960s and late-1970s), (b) the filler particles (between the late-1970s and mid-2000s) and, recently, (c) the resin matrix (between the mid-2000s and mid-2010s).

Improvements in resin composite technology have made possible a wide variety of additional applications, particularly in cosmetic dentistry (e.g., closing diastemas, transforming conoid teeth) and esthetic dental restoration with minimal loss of dental tissues [4]. With these advances has come a greater demand for esthetic-related treatment, which has guided the development of dental materials in recent years. For example, resin composites with different degrees of opacity [5] and simplified optical characteristics facilitate improved clinician ability to match the resin composite to the natural teeth, as is seen in universal color system technologies [6].

While the aforementioned advancements have allowed for greater clinical applications, over time resin composite restorations experience deterioration of texture and gloss as a result of a complex degradation process [7] (Figs. 9.1–9.3). While early in the development of dental technologies the primary goal was to achieve a restoration that was minimally resistant to wear and mechanical forces, currently the major challenge is the search for maintenance of the esthetic components of dental materials. This chapter will address intrinsic and extrinsic factors associated with resin composite discoloration, with the goal of reducing the need for early replacement.

9.1.1 Discoloration Due to Intrinsic Factors

9.1.1.1 Monomers

The color changes arising from the intrinsic processes of resin composites are commonly associ-

L. F. J. Schneider (✉)
School of Dentistry, Federal Fluminense University, Niterói, RJ, Brazil

Veiga de Almeida University, Rio de Janeiro, RJ, Brazil
e-mail: lfjschneider@id.uff.br

L. M. A. Cavalcante
School of Dentistry, Federal Fluminense University, Niterói, RJ, Brazil
e-mail: larissacavalcante@id.uff.br

D. Oliveira (ed.), *Color Science and Shade Selection in Operative Dentistry*,
https://doi.org/10.1007/978-3-030-99173-9_9

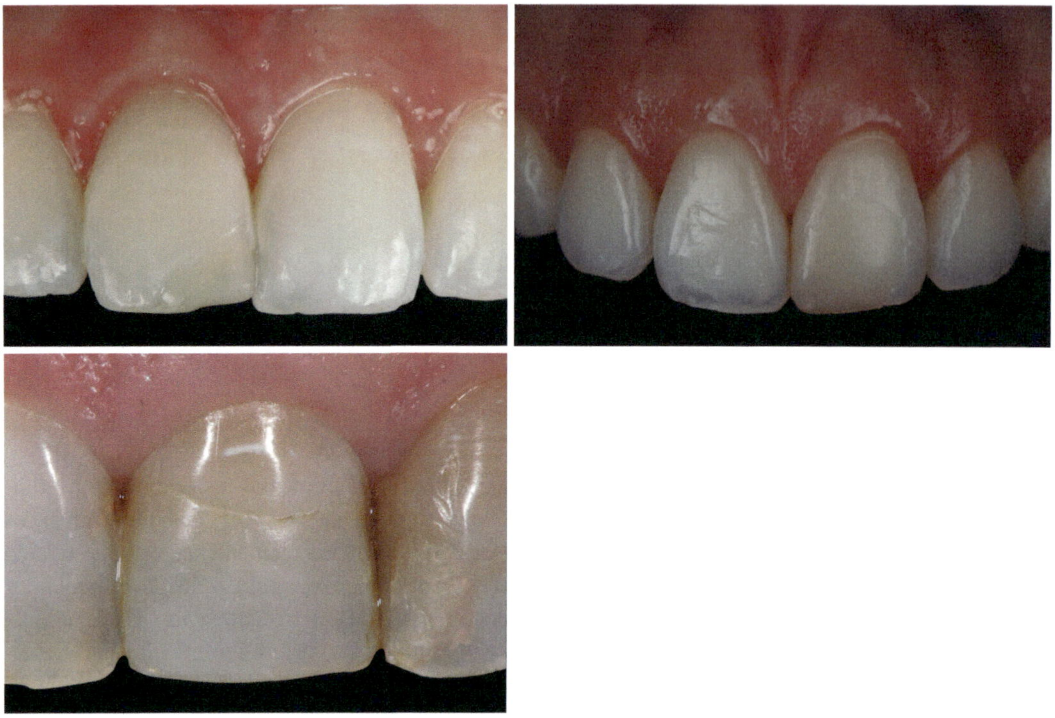

Figs. 9.1–9.3 Resin composite restorations degraded at different levels

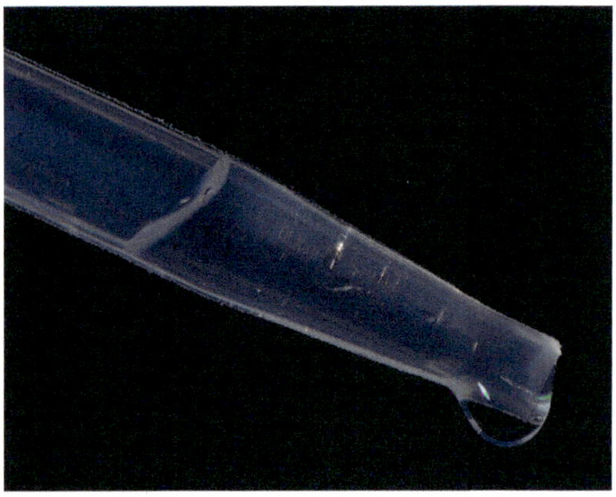

Fig. 9.4 BisGMA:TEGDMA (50:50 et%) monomer blend freshly removed from the bottle (Photography courtesy of Dr. Dayane Oliveira)

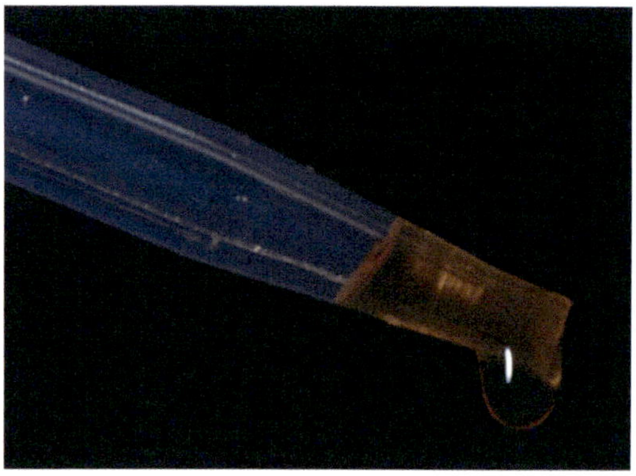

Fig. 9.5 BisGMA:TEGDMA (50:50 et%) monomer blend exposed to ambient light and air for 6 months at room temperature (Photography courtesy of Dr. Dayane Oliveira)

ated with the curing initiator system. Chemical alterations in the resin matrix can generate a yellowing effect in restorations, primarily due to the possible degradation of carbon–carbon double bonds in the unreacted monomers (Figs. 9.4 and 9.5) [8].

Thus, the chemical structure of the monomer and the physical characteristics of the three-dimensional polymeric structure are factors that have been shown to influence the optical characteristics of composites [9]. Multiple studies have reported that vinyl-groups can react with oxygen to form pigmented peroxides, a process that is accelerated by UV irradiation [10]. In this way, the composition of the resin matrix may influence physical property degradation and color stability of dental resin composites. Fonseca et al.

[11] investigated the influence of monomers regularly used in commercial resin composite formulations on the degree of conversion, water sorption, water solubility, and optical properties and found that all composites showed statistically significant differences in color stability after water aging. After 2 months in water storage, composites formulated with traditional base monomers (BisGMA, BisEMA, and UDMA) presented ΔE values lower than 3.3, a clinically acceptable value [12]. The lowest ΔE values were achieved by the base monomer BisEMA (1.0 ± 0.2), followed by UDMA (1.4 ± 0.2) and BisGMA (2.5 ± 0.5).

9.1.1.2 Photoinitiator System

The influence of the photoinitiator system on color change in resin composite restoration is a recurrent theme and has consistently affected the development of composite materials. Resin composites emerged for clinical use as self-curing systems that require the mixture of two pastes, which hinders the homogeneity of the components and often causes the problematic incorporation of bubbles into the mixture. Moreover, a significant level of amines is required for the polymerization process. According to Ruyter et al. [13] the unreacted amine components remain active in the polymeric network and can react with atmospheric oxygen or other aromatic compounds and increase the absorption of visible light. As a result, a significant color change can occur during the restoration.

In order to overcome this drawback, photoactivated systems using ultraviolet (UV) energy were developed. This evolution was a significant technological breakthrough as it also allowed clinicians to control working time. However, systems activated by UV-light have a low curing depth due to the thickness of the materials and high concentration of inorganic fillers. In addition, the use of ionizing radiation can cause a number of health problems for both the patient and the operator. Thus, it became necessary to search for an efficient and biologically safe photoinitiator system.

In 1971, Dart and Nemmeck [14], researchers at Imperial Chemical Industries, patented a system based on the use of an alpha-diketone as a composite component capable of absorbing light in the visible spectrum. Since then, camphorquinone has been used in the formulation of the vast majority of dental adhesives, restorative composites, and luting agents available on the dental market worldwide (Fig. 9.6). When irradiated by blue light, this molecule enters into an excitatory stage and, upon meeting an amine-type co-initiator (Fig. 9.7), abstracts a hydrogen atom from it and generates aminoalkyl radicals, which are then responsible for the chain polymerization process [15].

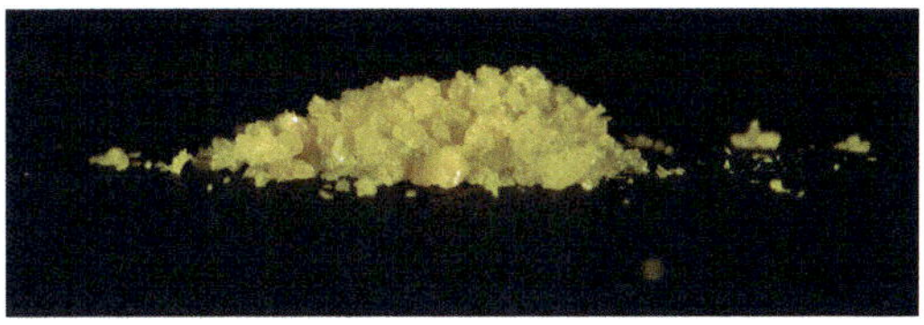

Fig. 9.6 Pure camphorquinone (CQ) (Photography courtesy of Dr. Dayane Oliveira)

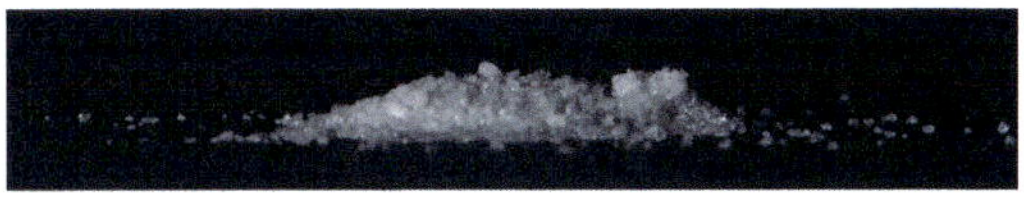

Fig. 9.7 Pure ethyl-4-dimethyl amine benzoate (Photography courtesy of Dr. Dayane Oliveira)

Although efficient and widely used for many years, there has been speculation regarding the potential drawbacks of the photoinitiator system based on the combination of camphorquinone and amine. Scientific articles commonly suggest that the concentration of camphorquinone in the resin composite formulation should be limited due to the intensity of the yellow hue it causes. However, it must be considered that when camphorquinone interacts with an efficient hydrogen donor, either an amine co-initiator or a specific monomer (such as UDMA, which will be discussed in the section on amine-free systems), a change in its molecular structure occurs causing a lightening, or photobleaching, effect [16].

The combination of camphorquinone and an amine is a binary system that depends on the interaction between two components to generate free radicals capable of initiating the chain-reaction polymerization process. Thus, the photobleaching process of camphorquinone is dependent on several factors. First, since the viscosity of the material can influence molecular diffusion, the photobleaching potential of camphorquinone may be affected by factors such as mass, temperature, and material composition. An additional factor, in theory, is the method by which the blue-light energy employed in the excitation process of camphorquinone is delivered. An activation process that employs a high amount of light energy in a short time due to the fast and cyclic interaction process between the camphorquinone and the amine may lose efficiency due to a lack of sufficient time for recombination. On the other hand, a low concentration of light energy delivery for a longer time may lose efficiency by increasing the viscosity of the material and consequently limiting the degree of monomeric conversion by reducing the molecular diffusion process. Thus, the counteracting effect of photobleaching may be limited, leading residual, unreacted camphorquinone molecules to produce a material with a yellow color shift [16].

In addition to the possible disadvantages associated with the use of camphorquinone, the need for an amine-type co-initiator system is also thought to be a limiting factor. Issues related to the toxic potential of these components aside, unreacted amines that are trapped inside the polymeric network can be sensitized by UV irradiation or chemical oxidation and generate compounds capable of causing color change that is perceptible to observers [13, 17–21]. As a result of multiple drawbacks to the camphorquinone and amine co-initiator system, alternative photoinitiator systems have been studied and developed in recent years.

Alternative Photoinitiator Systems

The partial or complete replacement of camphorquinone by other components is not new in research and innovation as well as commercially available clinical applications. In the late-1990s, for example, due to the popularization of tooth whitening, the company Bisco launched the Pyramid Enamel Neutral resin that comprised a photoinitiator system based entirely on the use of monoacylphosphine oxide (TPO), which is efficiently activated by halogen light sources and could, in theory, be used for formulations intended for highly whitened teeth or those treated with bleaching agents [22]. However, this system fell into disuse due to the development of exclusively blue diode (LED) light sources, which do not activate compounds that have maximum light absorption at wavelengths below blue [23]. With an increasing availability of LED light sources capable of emitting light at more than one wavelength, research on alternative non-camphorquinone photoactivator systems began again, with special attention paid to the possibility of enhancing the color stability of restorative materials.

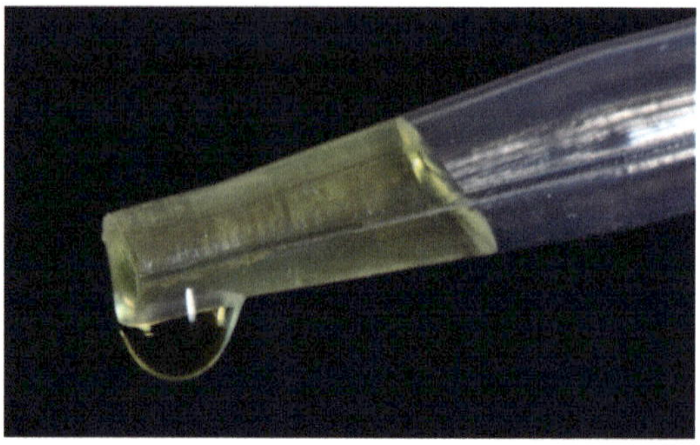

Fig. 9.8 Pure 1-phenyl-1,2-propanedione (PPD) (Photography courtesy of Dr. Dayane Oliveira)

The use of 1-phenyl-1,2-propanedione (PPD) was proposed by Park et al. [24]. According to the authors, this component had the potential to reduce the color change limitations associated with photoactivated resin composites (Fig. 9.8). However, no improvement in the photobleaching effect was detected when PPD was compared to camphorquinone after photoactivation [17, 18]. Schneider et al. [17] determined the polymerization potential and the yellowing effect of resin composites formulated with PPD, camphorquinone, or camphorquinone/PPD at different concentrations and found that the use of PPD did not reduce yellowing and also reduced surface hardness. Later, the same research group evaluated the effect of amine ethyl 4-dimethylaminobenzoate (EDMAB) ratio on the curing behavior, degradation resistance, and color change over time in experimental resin composites formulated with camphorquinone, PPD, and camphorquinone/PPD and found that the use of PPD did not reduce yellowing and negatively affected hardness [18]. De Oliveira et al. [25] studied the influence of PPD on yellowing and chemico-mechanical properties of experimental resin composites photoactivated by light curing and found that PPD alone did not achieve satisfactory results when compared to camphorquinone and camphorquinone/PPD. Furthermore, though there was a statistically significant reduction in the yellowing effect (CIELab parameters), the mean values were similar and only a small effect was detected in the final esthetic appearance.

Phosphine oxides are among the most researched alternative photoinitiator systems in dentistry. Several studies involving experimental resin composites have been performed using the ohotoinitiators bysacylphosphine oxide (BAPO) and TPO [23, 26–31] (Figs. 9.9 and 9.10). Studies have found that the use of TPO, alone or with camphorquinone, promoted less yellowing and improved color stability in restorative materials [27, 30, 32]. Although research on novel photoinitiator systems should be encouraged in the search for improved color stability, the traditional system based on the joint use of camphorquinone and amines continues to be a reliable formulation for dental composites [33]. In fact, some studies indicate that systems using camphorquinone and amines maintain better color stability over time than materials formulated with BAPO and TPO [34, 35]. Furthermore, the use of alternative photoinitiators with light absorption peaks located in shorter wavelengths negatively impacts the depth of polymerization of resin composites [19].

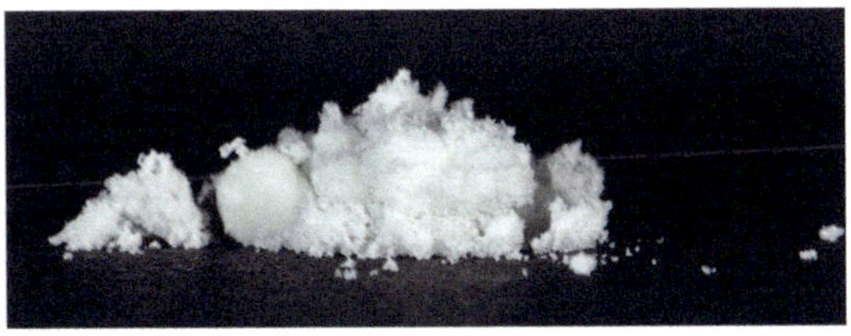

Fig. 9.9 Bysacylphosphine oxide (BAPO) (Photography courtesy of Dr. Dayane Oliveira)

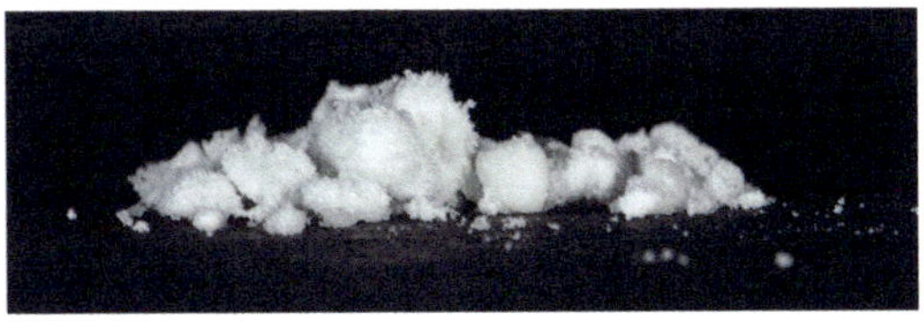

Fig. 9.10 Monoacylphosphine oxide (TPO) (Photography courtesy of Dr. Dayane Oliveira)

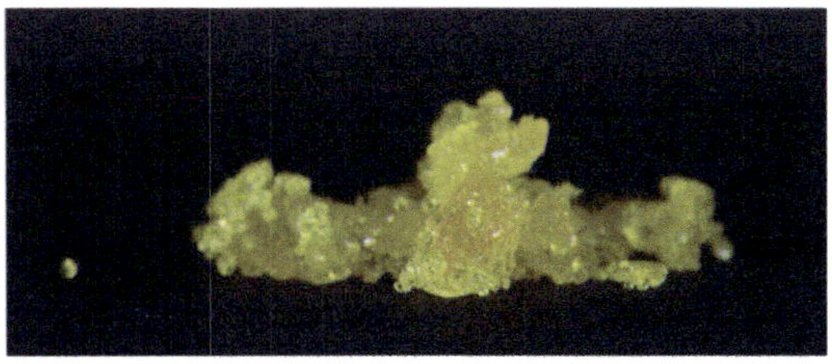

Fig. 9.11 Ivocerin™* (Ivoclar Vivadent). (*Photography courtesy of Dr. Dayane Oliveira, Dr. Mateus Rocha and Dr. Jean-François Roulet. *Kindly donated by Ivoclar Vivadent*)

The possibility of using germanium derivatives as a substitute for camphorquinone and amines has been studied and composites with these components are commercially available in dental materials under the registered name Ivocerin™ (Fig. 9.11) [35–37]. When employed in experimental composites, the germanium derivatives benzoyltrimethylgermane (BTMGe) and dibenzoyldiethylgermane (DBDEGe) showed higher color stability than materials formulated with a camphorquinone and amine-based system when exposed to UV irradiation [36]. However, in a study conducted with resin composites available for clinical use, Salgado et al. [35] found that resins formulated with the Ivocerin system showed the highest color variation after accelerated degradation testing by storage in water and coffee.

Another strategy that has been evaluated is the use of systems, with or without camphorquinone, omitting amine co-initiators not only to improve color stability but also to eliminate a component that is commonly associated with toxicity [38]. Asmussen et al. [16] found that camphorquinone oxidizes UDMA monomer and that the radicals derived from the UDMA monomer via hydrogen abstraction are highly reactive toward double bonds, achieving a similar level of double-bond conversion. The use of iodonium salts has been considered as a total or partial substitute for amine components and has shown interesting results in experimental resin composites [39, 40]. Very recently, sulfinates and sulfonates were evaluated as total replacements for amine components and produced materials with high polymerization ability and color stability [40]. The same research group has designed and tested alternative hydrogen donors for camphorquinone and found excellent photobleaching effects and color stability [41–43].

Amine-free materials are currently available for clinicians in the form of dual-cure resin cement and have demonstrated superior color stability compared to traditional cement that is formulated with high concentrations of amine components [44]. In this study, however, it was evident that other factors can have a more significant effect on color stability, including the amount of filler present in the system. One must also consider that commercially available materials employ UV-light stabilizers, which have an excellent ability to reduce the potential discoloration caused by the amine components.

9.1.2 Discoloration Due to Extrinsic Factors

The scientific literature on extrinsic factors associated with color change in resin composites commonly involves the long-term degradation process associated with pigment absorption. Color changes can be caused by the absorption of solvents of the organic matrix and/or the increased surface roughness that occurs for a number of reasons. However, it is necessary to consider that a series of events carried out during clinical practice can be instrumental in the maintenance of optical characteristics in the long term. For this reason, this section will address the extrinsic factors, separated into immediate (originating from clinical practice) and long-term factors, associated with material degradation.

9.1.3 Clinical-Related Factors

9.1.3.1 Material Selection

A wide variety of resin composites that produce excellent functional and esthetic results are available to clinicians. However, one must be aware that the selection of the material may affect the color stability of the restoration. Studies have shown that lighter and more translucent resins are associated with greater color change [35, 45, 46].

9.1.3.2 Material Handling

Although resin composites may inherently contain small amounts of micro-bubbles due to the manufacturing process [47], it is during the manipulation of the composite that the highest risk of introduction of large amounts of air inside the material occurs. This not only causes structural defects and subsequent mechanical failure but also reduces the polymerization potential and acts as a reservoir for pigment accumulation by absorption (which will be discussed in the following sections). Thus, the clinician should be aware that the maintenance of the optical properties of the restorative material is affected by the manner in which each resin increment is manipulated (Fig. 9.12).

During the process of sculpting the restoration, an increase in the viscosity of the material, and consequently the inclusion of air bubbles, may occur due to exposure of the material to light. For this reason, the clinician must avoid exposing the increments for prolonged periods to ambient light or worse, to light from the reflector.

Modeling liquids are commonly employed in clinical practice to improve the sculptability of restorative materials (Fig. 9.13). Several studies have been conducted to determine whether this practice has any impact (positive or negative) on

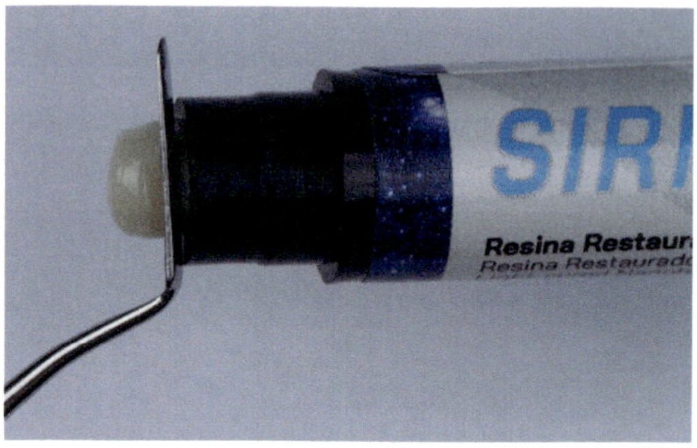

Fig. 9.12 Increment of resin composite correctly removed from the syringe

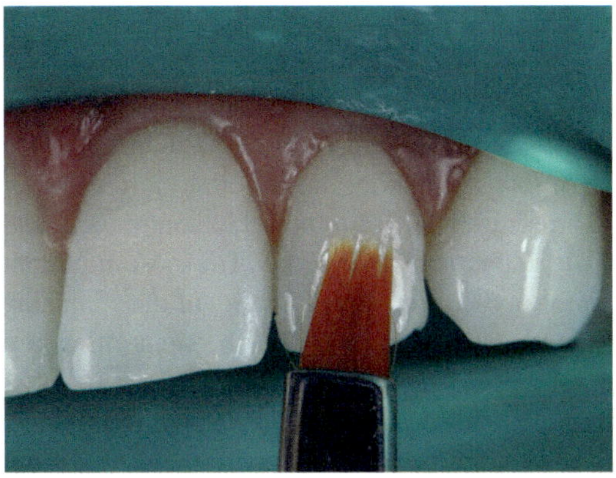

Fig. 9.13 Brush impregnated with modeling liquid to manipulate the increment with composite resin

the physicochemical properties of resin composites, with particular emphasis on optical properties. However, the results of these laboratory studies are limited due to a lack of standardization of either the evaluation processes, materials or treatments performed [48–55]. Considering the available literature, hydrophobicity appears to affect the efficacy of the modeling agent [56]. That is, an undesirable effect is more likely in cases where hydrophilic modeling agents such as simplified adhesives are used.

9.1.3.3 Photoactivation

The photoactivation process is directly associated with maintaining the esthetic aspects of resin composite restorations over time [57]. A higher degree of material conversion leads to lower concentrations of residual monomers susceptible to leaching processes and higher resistance to solvent penetration [58]. Thus, the more efficient the activation process of the material is, the more efficient the establishment of covalent bonds between the resin matrix with the silane and filler particles will be [59]. Furthermore, an efficient activation process is fundamental for the correct photobleaching effect of the camphorquinone and amine system [60].

9.1.3.4 Finishing and Polishing Procedures

The finishing and polishing steps are fundamental not only for the maintenance of color stability but also for the longevity of restorations performed with resin composite [61, 62]. In addition to promoting a smooth surface, which hinders pigment accumulation and abrasiveness, the finishing and polishing steps are responsible for removing the oxygen-inhibited layer. Failure to perform these steps, or inaccessibility of cutting or abrasion instruments to specific areas of the restoration, will cause a thin layer of the unpolymerized material to be directly exposed to a series of processes responsible for accelerated deterioration or pigmentation [63]. One caution that needs to be heeded is that rotary instruments should be used in conjunction with lubricants, as the resin matrix can degrade if elevated above 200 °C in finishing and polishing procedures [59].

9.1.4 Material-Related Factors

9.1.4.1 Degradation Process of the Resin Matrix

It should be noted that the polymerization process of composite materials takes place under extremely challenging conditions. The presence of oxygen from the environment, low atmospheric pressure, low ambient temperature, high material viscosity, and short time-limit to perform the tasks make it difficult to achieve a complete polymerization process. Thus, the monomers are never fully converted. Furthermore, when exposed to the oral environment, the resin matrix comes into contact with a series of agents, primarily saliva, which can act as solvents to leach the unreacted molecules and penetrate between the polymeric mesh formed, causing its separation and swelling and leaving the material softer and less resistant to wear [64]. Specific enzymes such as esterases can break the ester-type bonds commonly found in resins, further weakening the material [59, 65].

Resin composites are formulated by ceramic particles that are treated with a bonding agent and kept together by an agglutinating agent, the resin matrix, which is usually formulated by methacrylate monomers. Among the most-used methacrylate monomers, both in research and industrial application, is bisphenol A-glycerolate dimethacrylate

(BisGMA), a high-viscosity monomer with a stiff, aromatic central core, which can form a strong polymer network when associated with diluent co-monomers, usually triethylene glycol dimethacrylate (TEGDMA). Other base monomers include UDMA and ethoxylated bisphenol A dimethacrylate (BisEMA). Many studies have been performed on the influence of monomer composition on numerous properties, though little consideration has been given to the effect of resin matrix composition on the optical properties of resin composites. Fonseca et al. [10] found that the use of BisEMA promoted less resin composite color change over time, which was likely associated with BisEMA's lower affinity to water and lower volumetric expansion [66].

Considering the facts mentioned above, the amount of resin matrix used plays a key role in the color stability of resin composites, with materials formulated with higher inorganic content showing less color change [47]. As a result, great effort has been made to increase the resistance of the resin matrix to degradation by using monomers free of ester components or antimicrobial agents [67, 68]. Unfortunately, the products that have been launched and made available for clinical use have not been shown in the research to be advantageous in maintaining optical properties [9, 47, 67].

9.1.4.2 Degradation Process of the Filler Particles

The content of inorganic fillers present in resin composite material is directly associated with its resistance to degradation [68–72]. Although occurring at a much lower rate than that of the resin matrix, the filler particles are also subject to degradation processes. Water present in saliva can break down the filler particle surface through the process of hydrolysis and cause subsequent component leaching. In glass particles, for example, sodium atoms are removed and penetration of hydrogen atoms by water molecules takes place. Since the hydrogen atoms are smaller in size than the sodium atoms, a stress phenomenon can occur and thus break the surface [59].

9.1.4.3 Degradation Process of the Silane Layer

Silane bonding agents act on the bonding process between the inorganic filler particles and the resin matrix, making the material more resistant to stress transfer from the occlusion process and to degradation by hydrolysis. The most important factor in determining the quality of the silanizing treatment is the thickness of the silane film. If a single silane layer sufficiently covers the filler particle and promotes a bond with the resin matrix, additional silane layers may promote a disorganized, brittle, and breakable layer [59]. Thus, recent studies have sought to better understand the effect of the silane layer on the degradation process and optical properties of dental composites [73]. Recently, specific components or treatments like thiourethane filler functionalization have been evaluated as substitutes to the traditional one [68, 74].

9.2 Methods to Minimize Discoloration

9.2.1 Oral Hygiene

As previously mentioned, color changes in resin composites can be caused both by clinician choices and practices and by degradation mechanisms inherent to the composition of the material. With this in mind, some methods can be employed to minimize discoloration caused by pigmentation.

The habit of oral hygiene is fundamental for the maintenance of both oral and general health, and thus should always be encouraged. By removing the biofilm that accumulates on both the dental structure and the restorative material, the patient is actively removing pigments left as a result of diet and/or habits. While studies are inconclusive regarding the effect of toothpaste or mouthwash on the degradation process of resin composites [75–80], it is up to the professional to guide the patient regarding the need to avoid overly abrasive toothpaste or brushes, which may cause excessive wear of both the tooth structure and the restored area when used incorrectly.

9.2.2 Periodic Professional Cleaning

Periodic appointments are important to monitor the patient's oral health and to check the condition of previously placed restorations. This may include occlusal adjustment, contouring, or the need for a one-time addition of resin composite. In these appointments, rotary instruments such as Robinson brushes, rubber cups, or specific jets are commonly employed so that effective cleaning can be accomplished in the upper and lower arches in a short period of time. Studies have been conducted to determine the effect of different cleaning methods, with special attention to those based on air-polishing powders, on the surface properties of resin composites. Sodium bicarbonate, glycine, and erythritol have been tested [80–85]. Despite conflicting results and dependence on the material being evaluated, some studies point to glycine as being less harmful to the surface of restorations [83, 86].

Yap et al. [81] evaluated the effect of different cleaning methods on the surface of multiple direct-use restorative materials and suggested that it may be necessary to perform repolishing of the restored surfaces due to a potential increase in roughness. Guller et al. [84] has provided similar guidance.

9.3 Methods to Correct Discoloration

9.3.1 Bleaching

Tooth whitening has become an increasingly accessible and routine practice in dental offices. Although proven safe, questions remain regarding the effect of bleaching agents on preexisting restorations. Thus, it is essential that patients and clinicians are aware of the unpredictable nature of whitening treatments. While it is not guaranteed that a bleaching treatment will cause a color discrepancy between the tooth and restoration, it is a possibility and thus necessary that the patient be informed that this may occur and that a subsequent replacement of the restoration(s) may be required for esthetic reasons. Furthermore, although a bleaching effect may occur on the restoration due to the removal of pigments deposited both on the external surface and inside the mass, studies indicate that there may be a subsequent increase in the darkening of the restoration due to an increase in its roughness after exposure to a bleaching gel [87–89]. Moraes et al. [90] raised the question regarding potential bleaching effects on the surface integrity of exposed substrates, particularly with regard to the application of a highly concentrated solution. Although direct clinical effects depend on the actual in vivo conditions, bleaching procedures should not be carried out indiscriminately when restorations are present.

9.3.2 Repolishing vs. Replacing

As seen throughout this chapter, resin composites undergo a constant degradation process in the oral environment that may vary in speed and intensity depending on aspects related to both the patient (behavioral, physiological) and the clinician. Thus, the decision regarding what should be done with a restoration over time needs to consider both the patient's wishes and the practitioner's experience. When considering an esthetically unsatisfactory restoration, it is essential to identify the source of the problem.

If the origin of the problem is staining due to external pigments (e.g., coffee, wine, etc.) accumulated on surfaces that have become rough over the years, it is likely that a finishing and repolishing procedure is sufficient to restore the minimum conditions necessary for this restoration to remain in the mouth [91]. Restorations made of resin composites formulated with small-sized filler particles are likely to obtain a bright and smooth aspect easily [10]. On the other hand, if the discoloration occurs uniformly throughout the restoration and at a rate that is different than the remaining tooth structure, the cause is likely intrinsic in origin, which would necessitate a complete replacement.

Material fracture and secondary caries comprise the primary causes of failure of resin composite restorations requiring replacement. Color change is little reported in the literature as a major cause of failure in long-term studies, though is slightly more significant in studies performed on anterior teeth [92]. However, it must be considered that the demand for direct and indirect restorations for esthetic purposes has become greater in recent years and continues to be on an upward trajectory. As such, it is essential that dentistry professionals be aware of the need for continued development of clinical practice and new materials to accommodate this increased demand.

References

1. Ferracane JL. Resin composite—state of the art. Dent Mater. 2011;27(1):29–38.
2. Bayne SC, Ferracane JL, Marshall GW, Marshall SJ, van Noort R. The evolution of dental materials over the past century: silver and gold to tooth color and beyond. J Dent Res. 2019;98(3):257–65.
3. Miletic V. Development of dental composites. In: Dental composite materials for direct restorations. Cham: Springer; 2018.
4. Blatz MB, Chiche G, Bahat O, Roblee R, Coachman C, Heymann HO. Evolution of aesthetic dentistry. J Dent Res. 2019;98(12):1294–304.
5. Ryan EA, Tam LE, McComb D. Comparative translucency of esthetic composite resin restorative materials. J Can Dent Assoc. 2010;76:a84.
6. de Abreu JLB, Sampaio CS, Benalcázar Jalkh EB, Hirata R. Analysis of the color matching of universal resin composites in anterior restorations. J Esthet Restor Dent. 2020;29:269. https://doi.org/10.1111/jerd.12659.
7. Lee YK, Lu H, Oguri M, Powers JM. Changes in gloss after simulated generalized wear of composite resins. J Prosthet Dent. 2005;94(4):370–6.
8. Ferracane JL, Moser JB, Greener EH. Ultraviolet light induced yellowing of dental restorative resins. J Prosthet Dent. 1985;54(4):485–7.
9. Fonseca AS, Gerhardt KM, Pereira GD, Sinhoreti MA, Schneider LF. Do new matrix formulations improve resin composite resistance to degradation processes? Braz Oral Res. 2013;27(5):410–6.
10. Kolbeck C, Rosentritt M, Lang R, Handel G. Discoloration of facing and restorative composites by UV-irradiation and staining food. Dent Mater. 2006;22(1):63–8.
11. Fonseca AS, Labruna Moreira AD, de Albuquerque PP, de Menezes LR, Pfeifer CS, Schneider LF. Effect of monomer type on the CC degree of conversion, water sorption and solubility, and color stability of model dental composites. Dent Mater. 2017;33(4):394–401.
12. Vichi A, Ferrari M, Davidson CL. Color and opacity variations in three different resin-based composite products after water aging. Dent Mater. 2004;20(6):530–4.
13. Ruyter IE, Nilner K, Moller B. Color stability of dental resin materials for crown and bridge veneers. Dent Mater. 1987;3(5):246–51.
14. Dart EC, Cantwell JB, Traynor JR, Jaworzyn JF, Nemcek J, (Invs.). Curable dental filling compositions. US-PS 4,110,184, Imperial Chemical Industries; 1978.
15. Morlet-Savary F, Klee JE, Pfefferkorn F, Fouassier JP, Lalevée J. The camphorquinone/amine and camphorquinone/amine/phosphine oxide derivative photoinitiating systems: overview, mechanistic approach, and role of the excitation light source. Macromol Chem Phys. 2015;216(22):2161–70.
16. Asmusen S, Arenas G, Cook WD, Vallo C. Photobleaching of camphorquinone during polymerization of dimethacrylate-based resins. Dent Mater. 2009;25(12):1603–11.
17. Schneider LF, Pfeifer CS, Consani S, Prahl SA, Ferracane JL. Influence of photoinitiator type on the rate of polymerization, degree of conversion, hardness and yellowing of dental resin composites. Dent Mater. 2008;24(9):1169–77.
18. Schneider LF, Cavalcante LM, Consani S, Ferracane JL. Effect of co-initiator ratio on the polymer properties of experimental resin composites formulated with camphorquinone and phenyl–propanedione. Dent Mater. 2009;25(3):369–75.
19. Schneider LF, Cavalcante LM, Prahl SA, Pfeifer CS, Ferracane JL. Curing efficiency of dental resin composites formulated with camphorquinone or trimethylbenzoyl-diphenyl-phosphine oxide. Dent Mater. 2012;28(4):392–7.
20. Brandt WC, Schneider LF, Frollini E, Correr-Sobrinho L, Sinhoreti MA. Effect of different photo-initiators and light curing units on degree of conversion of composites. Braz Oral Res. 2010;24(3):263–70.
21. de Oliveira DC, Ayres AP, Rocha MG, Giannini M, Puppin Rontani RM, Ferracane JL, Sinhoreti MA. Effect of different in vitro aging methods on color stability of a dental resin-based composite using CIELAB and CIEDE2000 color-difference formulas. J Esthet Restor Dent. 2015;27(5):322–30.
22. Brandt WC, Consani S, Sinhoreti MAC, Cavalcante LMA, Schneider LF. Degree of conversion and crosslink density of resin composites formulated with different photoinitiators. RFO. 2009;14(3):239–45.
23. Moszner N, Salz U. Recent developments of new components for dental adhesives and composites. Macromol Mater Eng. 2007;292(3):245–71.

24. Park YJ, Chae KH, Rawls HR. Development of a new photoinitiation system for dental light-cure composite resins. Dent Mater. 1999;15(2):120–7.
25. de Oliveira DC, Souza-Junior EJ, Dobson A, Correr AR, Brandt WC, Sinhoreti MA. Evaluation of phenyl–propanedione on yellowing and chemical–mechanical properties of experimental dental resin-based materials. J Appl Oral Sci. 2016;24(6):555–60.
26. Leprince JG, Hadis M, Shortall AC, Ferracane JL, Devaux J, Leloup G, Palin WM. Photoinitiator type and applicability of exposure reciprocity law in filled and unfilled photoactive resins. Dent Mater. 2011;27(2):157–64.
27. Albuquerque PP, Moreira AD, Moraes RR, Cavalcante LM, Schneider LF. Color stability, conversion, water sorption and solubility of dental composites formulated with different photoinitiator systems. J Dent. 2013;41(3):e67–72.
28. Randolph LD, Palin WM, Watts DC, Genet M, Devaux J, Leloup G, Leprince JG. The effect of ultra-fast photopolymerisation of experimental composites on shrinkage stress, network formation and pulpal temperature rise. Dent Mater. 2014;30(11):1280–9.
29. Randolph L, Leloup G, Palin WM, Leprince JG. Trapped radicals in Lucirin-TPO vs camphorquinone-based dental composites. Dent Mater. 2013;29:45–50.
30. Salgado VE, Borba MM, Cavalcante LM, Moraes RR, Schneider LF. Effect of photoinitiator combinations on hardness, depth of cure, and color of model resin composites. J Esthet Restor Dent. 2015;27(1):S41–8.
31. Bertolo MV, Moraes RC, Pfeifer C, Salgado VE, Correr AR, Schneider LF. Influence of photoinitiator system on physical–chemical properties of experimental self-adhesive composites. Braz Dent J. 2017;28(1):35–9.
32. Salgado VE, Albuquerque PP, Cavalcante LM, Pfeifer CS, Moraes RR, Schneider LF. Influence of photoinitiator system and nanofiller size on the optical properties and cure efficiency of model composites. Dent Mater. 2014;30(10):e264–71.
33. Albuquerque PP, Bertolo ML, Cavalcante LM, Pfeifer C, Schneider LF. Degree of conversion, depth of cure, and color stability of experimental dental composite formulated with camphorquinone and phenanthrenequinone photoinitiators. J Esthet Restor Dent. 2015;27(1):S49–57.
34. de Oliveira DC, Rocha MG, Gatti A, Correr AB, Ferracane JL, Sinhoret MA. Effect of different photoinitiators and reducing agents on cure efficiency and color stability of resin-based composites using different LED wavelengths. J Dent. 2015;43(12):1565–72.
35. Salgado VE, Rego GF, Schneider LF, Moraes RR, Cavalcante LM. Does translucency influence cure efficiency and color stability of resin-based composites? Dent Mater. 2018;34(7):957–66.
36. Moszner N, Fischer UK, Ganster B, Liska R, Rheinberger V. Benzoyl germanium derivatives as novel visible light photoinitiators for dental materials. Dent Mater. 2008;24(7):901–7.
37. Ganster B, Fischer UK, Moszner N, Liska R. New photocleavable structures. IV. Acylgerman based photoinitiator for visible light curing. Macromol Rapid Commun. 2008;29(1):57–62.
38. Vasquez B, Levenfeld B, San RJ. Role of amine activators on the curing parameters, properties and toxicity of acrylic bone cements. Polym Int. 1998;46:241–50.
39. Shin DH, Rawls HR. Degree of conversion and color stability of the light curing resin with new photoinitiator systems. Dent Mater. 2009;25(8):1030–8.
40. Kirschner J, Szillat F, Bouzrati-Zerelli M, Becht JM, Klee JE, Lalevée J. Sulfinates and sulfonates as high performance co-initiators in CQ based systems: towards aromatic amine-free systems for dental restorative materials. Dent Mater. 2020;36(2):187–96.
41. Sprick E, Graff B, Becht JM, Tigges T, Neuhaus K, Weber C, Lalevee J. New bio-sourced hydrogen donors as high performance coinitiators and additives for CQ-based systems: toward aromatic amine-free photoinitiating systems. Eur Polym J. 2020;134:109794.
42. Sprick E, Becht JM, Tigges T, Neuhaus K, Weber C, Lalevee J. Hydrogen donors to replace aromatic amine based photoinitiating systems. Nano Select. 2020;1:382–7.
43. Sprick E, Becht JM, Graff B, Salomon JP, Tigges T, Weber C, Lalevée J. New hydrogen donors for amine-free photoinitiating systems in dental materials. Dent Mater. 2021;37(3):382–90.
44. Schneider LFJ, Ribeiro RB, Liberato WF, Salgado VE, Moraes RR, Cavalcante LM. Curing potential and color stability of different resin-based luting materials. Dent Mater. 2020;36(10):e309–15.
45. Uchida H, Vaidyanathan J, Viswanadhan T, Vaidyanathan TK. Color stability of dental composites as a function of shade. J Prosthet Dent. 1998;79(4):372–7.
46. Piccoli YB, Lima VP, Basso GR, Salgado VE, Lima GS, Moraes RR. Optical stability of high-translucency resin-based composites. Oper Dent. 2019;44(5):536–44.
47. Cavalcante LM, Schneider LF, Hammad M, Watts DC, Silikas N. Degradation resistance of ormocer- and dimethacrylate-based matrices with different filler contents. J Dent. 2012;40(1):86–90.
48. Valentini F, Oliveira SG, Guimarães GZ, Barbosa RP, Moraes RR. Effect of surface sealant on the color stability of composite resin restorations. Braz Dent J. 2011;22(5):365–8.
49. Tuncer S, Demirci M, Tiryaki M, Unlü N, Uysal Ö. The effect of a modeling resin and thermocycling on the surface hardness, roughness, and color of different resin composites. J Esthet Restor Dent. 2013;25(6):404–19.
50. Münchow EA, Sedrez-Porto JA, Piva E, Pereira-Cenci T, Cenci MS. Use of dental adhesives as modeler liquid of resin composites. Dent Mater. 2016;32(4):570–7.
51. Sedrez-Porto JA, Münchow EA, Brondani LP, Cenci MS, Pereira-Cenci T. Effects of modeling liquid/resin

and polishing on the color change of resin composite. Braz Oral Res. 2016;30(1).
52. Araujo FS, Barros MC, Santana ML, Oliveira LS, Silva PF, Lima GS, Faria-E-Silva AL. Effects of adhesive used as modeling liquid on the stability of the color and opacity of composites. J Esthet Restor Dent. 2018;30(5):427–33.
53. Brooksbank A, Owens BM, Phebus JG, Blen BJ, Wasson W. Surface sealant effect on the color stability of a composite resin following ultraviolet light artificial aging. Oper Dent. 2019;44(3):322–30.
54. Rizzante FA, Bombonatti JS, Vasconcelos L, Porto TS, Teich S, Mondelli RF. Influence of resin-coating agents on the roughness and color of composite resins. J Prosthet Dent. 2019;122(3):332.e1–5.
55. Cortopassi LS, Shimokawa CA, Willers AE, Sobral MA. Surface roughness and color stability of surface sealants and adhesive systems applied over a resin-based composite. J Esthet Restor Dent. 2020;32(1):64–72.
56. Sedrez-Porto JA, Münchow EA, Cenci MS, Pereira-Cenci T. Translucency and color stability of resin composite and dental adhesives as modeling liquids—a 1-year evaluation. Braz Oral Res. 2017;31:e54.
57. Janda R, Roulet J-F, Latta M, Kaminsky M, S R. Effect of exponential polymerization on color stability of resin-based filling materials. Dent Mater. 2007;23(6):696–704.
58. da Silva Alberton V, da Silva Alberton S, Pecho OE, Bacchi A. Influence of composite type and light irradiance on color stability after immersion in different beverages. J Esthet Restor Dent. 2018;30(5):390–6.
59. Söderholm KJ. Degradation mechanisms of dental resin composites. In: Eliades G, Eliades T, Brantley WA, Watts DC, editors. Dental materials in vivo: aging and related phenomena. New Malden: Quintessence; 2003.
60. Brackett MG, Brackett WW, Browning WD, Rueggeberg FA. The effect of light curing source on the residual yellowing of resin composites. Oper Dent. 2007;32(5):443–50.
61. Egilmez F, Ergun G, Cekic-Nagas I, Vallittu PK, Lassila LV. Short and long term effects of additional post curing and polishing systems on the color change of dental nano-composites. Dent Mater J. 2013;32(1):107–14.
62. Duc O, Bella ED, Krejci I, Betrisey E, Abdelaziz M, Ardu S. Staining susceptibility of resin composite materials. Am J Dent. 2019;32(1):39–42.
63. Schroeder T, Silva TB, Basso GR, Franco MC, Maske TT, Cenci MS. Factors affecting the color stability and staining of esthetic restorations. Odontology. 2019;107(4):507–12.
64. Moraes RR, Marimon JL, Schneider LF, Sinhoreti MA, Correr-Sobrinho L, Bueno M. Effects of 6 months of aging in water on hardness and surface roughness of two microhybrid dental composites. J Prosthodont. 2008;17(4):323–6.
65. Ferracane J. Hygroscopic and hydrolytic effects in dental polymer networks. Dent Mater. 2006;22(3):211–22.
66. Sideridou ID, Karabela MM, Vouvoudi EC. Volumetric dimensional changes of dental light-cured dimethacrylate resins after sorption of water or ethanol. Dent Mater. 2008;24(8):1131–6.
67. Schneider LF, Cavalcante LM, Silikas N, Watts DC. Degradation resistance of silorane, experimental ormocer and dimethacrylate resin-based dental composites. J Oral Sci. 2011;53(4):413–9.
68. Fugolin AP, Pfeifer CS. New resins for dental composites. J Dent Res. 2017;96(10):1085–91.
69. Cavalcante LM, Masouras M, Watts DC, Pimenta LA, Silikas N. Effect of nanofillers' size on surface properties after toothbrush abrasion. Am J Dent. 2009;22(1):60–4.
70. Kaizer MR, Oliveira-Ogliari A, Cenci MS, Opdam NJ, Moraes RR. Do nanofill or submicron composites show improved smoothness and gloss? A systematic review of in vitro studies. Dent Mater. 2014;30(4):e41–78.
71. Salgado VE, Cavalcante LM, Silikas N, Schneider LF. The influence of nanoscale inorganic content over optical and surface properties of model composites. J Dent. 2013;41(5):e45–53.
72. Salgado VE, Cavalcante LM, Moraes RR, Davis HB, Ferracane JL, Schneider LF. Degradation of optical and surface properties of resin-based composites with distinct nanoparticle sizes but equivalent surface area. J Dent. 2017;59:48–53.
73. Cavalcante LM, Ferraz LG, Antunes KB, Garcia IM, Schneider LFJ, Collares FM. Silane content influences physicochemical properties in nanostructured model composites. Dent Mater. 2021;37(2):e85–93.
74. Cavalcante LM, Ramos AB, Silva DC, Alves GG, Antunes KB, Pfeifer CS, Schneider LFJ. Thiourethane-functionalized fillers: biological properties and degradation resistance. Braz Oral Res. 2021;35:e018.
75. Festuccia MS, Garcia LD, Cruvinel DR, Pires-De-Souza FD. Color stability, surface roughness and microhardness of composites submitted to mouth rinsing action. J Appl Oral Sci. 2012;20(2):200–5.
76. Roselino LM, Cruvinel DR, Chinelatti MA, Pires-de-Souza FCP. Effect of brushing and accelerated ageing on color stability and surface roughness of composites. J Dent. 2013;41(5):e54–61.
77. Lai G, Zhao L, Wang J, Kunzelmann KH. Surface properties and color stability of dental flowable composites influenced by simulated tooth brushing. Dent Mater J. 2018;37(5):717–24.
78. Mathias-Santamaria IF, Roulet JF. The effect of diamond toothpastes on surface gloss of resin composites. Am J Dent. 2019;32(4):169–73.
79. de Moraes Rego Roselino L, Tirapelli C, de Carvalho Panzeri Pires-de-Souza F. Randomized clinical study of alterations in the color and surface roughness of

dental enamel brushed with whitening toothpaste. J Esthet Restor Dent. 2018;30(5):383–9.
80. de Moraes Rego Roselino L, Tonani Torrieri R, Sbardelotto C, Alves Amorim A, Noronha Ferraz de Arruda C, Tirapelli C, de Carvalho Panzeri Pires-de-Souza F. Color stability and surface roughness of composite resins submitted to brushing with bleaching toothpastes: an in situ study. J Esthet Restor Dent. 2019;31(5):486–92.
81. Yap AU, Wu SS, Chelvan S, Tan ES. Effect of hygiene maintenance procedures on surface roughness of composite restoratives. Oper Dent. 2005;30(1):99–104.
82. Pelka MA, Altmaier K, Petschelt A, Lohbauer U. The effect of air-polishing abrasives on wear of direct restoration materials and sealants. J Am Dent Assoc. 2010;141(1):63–70.
83. Giacomelli L, Salerno M, Derchi G, Genovesi A, Paganin PP, Covani U. Effect of air polishing with glycine and bicarbonate powders on a nanocomposite used in dental restorations: an in vitro study. Int J Periodontics Restor Dent. 2011;31(5):e51–6.
84. Güler AU, Duran I, Yücel AÇ, Ozkan P. Effects of air-polishing powders on color stability of composite resins. J Appl Oral Sci. 2011;19(5):505–10.
85. Amari Y, Takamizawa T, Kawamoto R, Namura Y, Murayama R, Yokoyama M, Tsujimoto A, Miyazaki M. Influence of one-step professional mechanical tooth cleaning pastes on surface roughness and morphological features of tooth substrates and restoratives. J Oral Sci. 2020;30:0420. https://doi.org/10.2334/josnusd.20-0420.
86. Janiszewska-Olszowska J, Drozdzik A, Tandecka K, Grocholewicz K. Effect of air-polishing on surface roughness of composite dental restorative material—comparison of three different air-polishing powders. BMC Oral Health. 2020;20(1):30.
87. Yu H, Pan X, Lin Y, Li Q, Hussain M, Wang Y. Effects of carbamide peroxide on the staining susceptibility of tooth-colored restorative materials. Oper Dent. 2009;34(1):72–82.
88. Della Bona A, Pecho OE, Ghinea R, Cardona JC, Paravina RD, Perez MM. Influence of bleaching and aging procedures on color and whiteness of dental composites. Oper Dent. 2019;44(6):648–58.
89. Vidal ML, Pecho OE, Xavier J, Della BA. Influence of the photoactivation distance on the color and whiteness stability of resin-based composite after bleaching and aging. J Dent. 2020;99:103408.
90. Moraes RR, Marimon JL, Schneider LF, Correr Sobrinho L, Camacho GB, Bueno M. Carbamide peroxide bleaching agents: effects on surface roughness of enamel, composite and porcelain. Clin Oral Investig. 2006;10(1):23–8.
91. Mundim FM, Garcia LF, Pires-de-Souza FCP. Effect of staining solutions and repolishing on color stability of direct composites. J Appl Oral Sci. 2010;18(3):249–54.
92. Demarco FF, Collares K, Coelho-de-Souza FH, Correa MB, Cenci MS, Moraes RR, Opdam NJ. Anterior composite restorations: a systematic review on long-term survival and reasons for failure. Dent Mater. 2015;31(10):1214–24.

Longevity of Resin Composite Restorations

10

Flávio Fernando Demarco, Luiz Alexandre Chisini, Marcos Britto Correa, Maximiliano Sérgio Cenci, and Rafael Ratto de Moraes

Composite resin restorations have been the first choice by clinicians and patients for direct anterior [1] and posterior restorations [2] mainly due to optical characteristics, high longevity, adhesive properties, and preservation of sound tooth structure [3, 4]. Resin composite restorations have presented a lower annual failure rate (AFR) ranging from 1 to 3% in posterior teeth and 1–5% in anterior teeth [5]. Recent publications have shown that this material can be used to rehabilitate severely worn teeth with acceptable clinical success, with AFR ranging from 0.4% for microhybrid composites to 26.3% for microfilled materials [6]. Similarly, a network meta-analysis found an AFR of 2.2% for use in large posterior restorations [7].

The main reasons for failure in posterior restorations, both in adults [8] and children [9], are fractures and secondary caries. It has been discussed that material properties had a minor effect on longevity. At the same time, clinical-related factors (such as the position of the tooth in the tooth arc and dental type), the operator (age, country of qualification, and employment status), patient (caries risk, bruxing habits, parafunction, esthetic demand), and socioeconomic status might play essential roles in the longevity of composites [10]. Tooth structure or composite fractures are important factors for restorations failure, while esthetic demands could account for restoration replacement in anterior teeth [11].

To improve dental restorations' longevity and under a minimally invasive dentistry philosophy, repair has been proposed as an interesting strategy over the replacement, avoiding the repetitive restorative cycle [12]. Removal of the sound dental structure occurs when the complete restoration is replaced. When the restoration needing replacement is near the vital pulp tissue, the risk of pulp exposure is elevated and can result in unnecessary endodontic treatments [13, 14]. Therefore, resin restorations can be repaired when a considerable part of restoration presents good condition to be maintained. Repair of defective restorations has exhibited good clinical performance, increasing dental restorations' longevity (Fig. 10.1) [10, 15] and displaying better cost-effectiveness than replacement [16]. In this chapter, we will discuss the longevity of esthetic composite restorations, the reasons for failure, and exploring the repair of defective restorations as a treatment option to the replacement.

10.1 Expectation vs. Reality

Resin composites have undergone constant development, becoming the most used direct restorative material [2], mainly because of their

F. F. Demarco (✉) · M. B. Correa · M. S. Cenci
R. R. de Moraes
Department of Restorative Dentistry, College of Dentistry, Federal University of Pelotas, Pelotas, RS, Brazil

L. A. Chisini
Department of Restorative Dentistry, College of Dentistry, Federal University of Juiz de Fora, Governador Valadares, MG, Brazil

D. Oliveira (ed.), *Color Science and Shade Selection in Operative Dentistry*,
https://doi.org/10.1007/978-3-030-99173-9_10

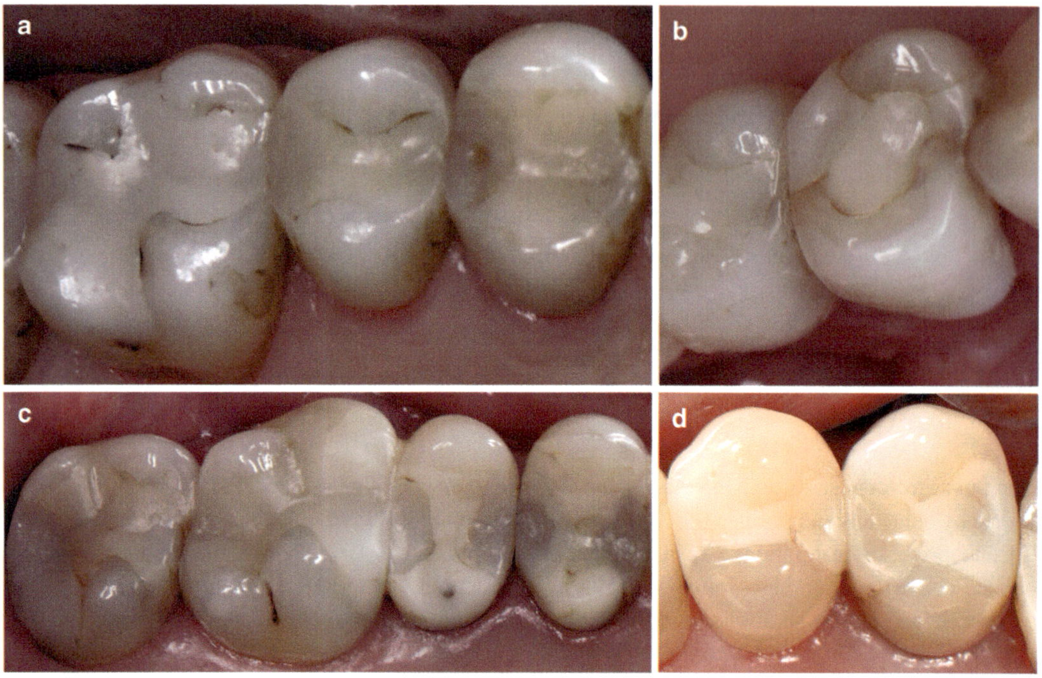

Fig. 10.1 Clinical phenotypes of resin composite restorations in posterior teeth after at least two decades of clinical service. In (**a**) and (**b**), the restorations show typical signs of aging including loss of anatomical form, surface and marginal staining, color instability, and wear. In (**c**), restorations were repaired and still presented good clinical performance after several years in the mouth. In (**d**), restorations were repaired and subjected to polishing, which removed the extrinsic staining and improved appearance. (*Photography courtesy of Dr. Paullo Rodolpho*)

esthetic properties, preservation of tooth structure, and the high success rates [3, 17]. Considering the results from clinical studies about the longevity of composite restorations, clinicians frequently expect a longevity of more than 20 years for their restorations. However, despite the excellent results showed in the literature, dentists should be aware that different aspects involving themselves, the tooth/cavity, and the patient can interfere with the durability of a restorations. The understanding of these factors can help professionals to predict better the probability of failure of a given restoration.

A vast number of systematic reviews have been published in recent literature presenting the AFR/success rate (SR) of resin composites [10, 11, 18–28] (Table 10.1). In general, the systematic reviews have presented similar results: AFR ranging from 1 to 3% in posterior teeth and from 1 to 5% in anterior teeth [5]. The AFR increases when endodontic treated teeth are investigated: ranging from 2 to 12.4% [10]. It is important to highlight that several systematic reviews are based exclusively on prospective clinical trials, including low-risk patients. On the other hand, practice-based studies have displayed AFR higher when patients with high risk are included [8, 35]. In 11 Dutch general practices, a Practice-Based Study evaluated 31,472 restorations observed an AFR of 7.8% at 2 years [35]. A similar practice-based retrospective study that assessed the survival of resin composite restorations in posterior teeth found that 30% of the restorations failed, of which 82% were found in patients with high-risk factors, being secondary caries the main reason for failure [8].

The expectation of longevity is often determined by empirical criteria or measures, such as the average age of a failed restoration. There are several factors associated with restorative failures that are important to be evaluated for each clinical situation and can more accurately predict the longevity of restorations. The clinician's expectations should be based on the assessment

Table 10.1 Results from systematic reviews on the clinical performance of resin composite restorations

Study	Tooth type	Factors associated with failure	Mains reason to failure	Follow-up (years)	AFR/survival proportion (SR)
Arbildo-Vega et al., 2020 [29]	Class I, II and V	NR	NR	0.5–10	NR
Veloso et al., 2019 [30]	Posterior (class I and II)	NR	Caries, fracture, sensitivity, anatomical shape, marginal discoloration	1–6	SP: 94.4% bulk-fill; 96.7% conventional composite
Azeem and Sureshbabu, 2018 [31]	Posterior (direct and indirect)	NR	NR	1–11	NR
Afrashtehfar et al., 2017 [18]	Posterior endodontically treated teeth	Number of restored surfaces, restorative material, and technique	NR	3–10	SP: 89.7% (3 years); 92.4% (5 years)
Afrashtehfar et al., 2017 [19]	Posterior	Number of restored surfaces	NR	3–6	SR: 50–100%
Ahmed and Murbay, 2016 [20]	Anterior (tooth wear)	Occlusal	Fractures of restoration	0.5–10	SR: >90% (2.5 years); 50% (5 years)
van de Sande et al., 2016 [28]	Posterior	Patient age, gender, caries risk, and parafunctional habits	Caries and fracture	3–21	AFR: 1.7–5.2% SP: 72–95%
Angeletaki et al., 2016 [21]	Posterior (inlay/onlay)	NR	Fracture and cohesive restoration failure	4.5–11	SR: 83.2% (5 years)
Moraschini et al., 2015 [26]	Posterior (class I and II)	NR	Fracture (tooth or restoration) and caries	1–10	AFR: 3.17%
Mesko et al., 2016 [6]	Several worn teeth	NR	NR	0.5–12	AFR: 0.4% (microhybrid); 26.3% (microfilled)
da Veiga et al., 2016 [24]	Posterior (class I and II)	None	Fracture (tooth or restoration)	2–11	NR
Demarco et al., 2015 [11]	Anterior (class III and IV, veneers and reanatomization)	Adhesive technique, composite resin, retreatment risk, and time required to build-up the restoration	Fracture of tooth/ restoration and esthetic qualities	3–17	AFR: 0–4.1% SR: 100% (3 years); 53.4% (15 years)
Heintze et al., 2015 [25]	Anterior (class III and IV, diastema closures)	Cavity type, restorative material, bonding strategy	Bulk fractures and caries	2–12	SP: 95% (10 years—class III) 90% (10 years—class IV)
Astvaldsdottir et al., 2015 [22]	Posterior	NR	Caries, fracture, and restoration loss	4–12	SP: 93% (4 years); 91 (5 years)
Opdam et al., 2014 [27]	Posterior (class I and II)	Patient caries risk, presence of lining cement, number of restored surfaces, composite filler loading	Caries and fracture (tooth or restoration)	6–22	AFR: 1.8% (5 years); 2.4% (10 years)
Rasines Alcaraz et al., 2014 [32]	Posterior	Restorative material	Caries, fracture, and restoration loss	5–7	NR

(continued)

Table 10.1 (continued)

Study	Tooth type	Factors associated with failure	Mains reason to failure	Follow-up (years)	AFR/survival proportion (SR)
Fron Chabouis et al., 2013 [33]	Posterior (inlays and onlays)	Restorative material (ceramic better than composite)	Fracture (tooth or restoration) and caries	3–10	SP: 73.7% for composite inlays
Heintze and Rousson, 2012 [34]	Posterior (class I and II)	Bonding strategy, restorative material, operative procedure	Bulk fractures and caries	2–9	SP: 90% (10 years)
Demarco et al., 2012 [10]	Posterior	Clinical, operator, patient, socioeconomic, material	Fracture (restoration or tooth) and secondary caries	5–22	AFR 1–3%

NR not reported, *AFR* annual failure rate, *SR* cumulative survival rate

of risk factors, which may help a more accurate estimate. Thus, when the restoration is placed on a patient with risk factors (sometimes more than one) it is expected that the durability of this restoration may be less than average observed. On the other hand, when few risk factors are found clinically, greater longevity can be expected. To predict better the likelihood of restoration failure and make the expectation closer to reality, we need to discuss the main factors associated with the failure of composite materials.

10.1.1 Long-Term Survival and Reasons for Failures

Data on composite resin restorations' survival have been widely explored for posterior teeth, while data of anterior teeth is more limited in the literature [11]. The main reasons for failure in posterior restorations seem to be secondary caries and the fracture of teeth/restorations [3, 26, 27] (Table 10.2). When high-risk patients are included, secondary caries commonly is reported as the main reason for restoration failure [8, 35, 51]. Fractures are frequently linked with premature or long-term (fatigue of material) failures, while caries is related to long-term follow-ups [52].

Fracture and esthetic demand have been reported as the main failure reasons for anterior esthetic restoration. Indeed, when the anterior restoration is placed for an esthetic reason, the likelihood main reason for failure will be related to esthetics (such as color match, anatomical form, or surface stain) [11]. Although direct comparisons between anterior and posterior restorations are not appropriate, in general, anterior restorations behave differently from posterior restorations, presenting reduced failures for "loss of restoration" or caries. At the same time, esthetic appearance plays a prominent role in the patient's desire to have a restoration replaced.

10.1.1.1 Dental Caries

Secondary caries are reported to be the main reason for restoration's failure. By definition, secondary or recurrent caries are "lesions at the margins of existing restorations" or "caries associated with restorations or sealants" (CARS) [53, 54]. It is important to note that restoring a tooth is not the definitive treatment for caries disease—but it may be a part of the treatment. To be clear, it is necessary to control all the etiological factors that are causing the disease [55]. The understanding of the causal factors for caries development and their respective control is necessary. As it is well-established, caries is a sugar-biofilm-dependent disease, and epidemiological studies have shown that sugar consumption in the life course is associated with caries lesions [56, 57]. In addition to diet, fluoride consumption, hygiene habits, socioeconomic factors, among others, are essential to be investigated and influence restoration's survival through secondary caries failures. Considering these aspects, it is possible to treat caries disease properly, preventing the occurrence of secondary caries.

The failure to interrupt the caries disease can contribute to the failure of the restoration [58]. After 18 years, a retrospective study found that 68.4% of failures were due to secondary caries [59]. Posterior restorations placed in children with high DMFT index displayed a high risk to

Table 10.2 Summary of main factors involved in longevity of composite restorations and their respective effect measures

Factor	Effect
Tooth type	– Molars present 2.3 times higher risk of failure than premolars [36] – Upper central incisors have 1.3 times higher risk of failure than lower lateral incisors [37]
Cavity size	– Each restored surface's addition leads to an increase of 40% in the risk of failure [38] – For premolars, each surface included in the restoration introduces an increase of 50% on the risk for failure, while for molars, this risk is increased by 24% for each surface [27]
Previous endodontic treatment	– Veneers made in non-vital teeth had a higher risk of failure (178% greater) over time compared to those made in vital teeth [39] – Endodontic treatment increases the risk of failure in posterior teeth (HR 25.3) [40]
Selective caries removal	– Selective caries removal does not affect the longevity of restorations, and due to the fact that it reduces the risk of pulp exposures, it should be chosen [41–43]
Substrate type	There is no consensus in the literature: – Higher AFR was observed for class II restorations with glass ionomer bases compared with restorations without a base material [38] – No significant differences were observed after 18 years of posterior composite survival with and without glass ionomer cement as a base [44]
Caries risk	– AFR was 4.2% in the high-risk group and 0.9% in the low caries risk group [45] – Presence of unsatisfactory restorations was 5.3 higher in children at high risk of caries in the permanent dentition than children classified at low risk [46]
Bruxism and/or parafunctional habits	– Restorations in individuals with high occlusal-stress presented 2.6 times higher risk for failure than individuals with no occlusal-stress [8]
Socioeconomic status	– Posterior restorations' failures are 2.2-fold more prevalent in low-income individuals [47]
Operator	– Important variations in the longevity of composite restorations were observed according to the dentist [48]
Material	– To observe the effect of materials properties on annual failure rates long periods are needed [5, 10, 17]
Esthetic demands	– Anterior restoration placed for esthetic reasons presents a higher likelihood to be changed due to esthetics-related factors such as color match, anatomical form, or surface stain [11]
Rubber dam isolation	– The use of rubber dam seems not to be decisively provided that good isolation with cotton and suction is achieved [49]
Enamel beveling	– Enamel beveling does not affect the clinical performance of the restoration [34]
Adhesive system	– Gold standard dental adhesive technique is the use of a mild two-step, a self-etch adhesive system with selective phosphoric acid enamel etching [50]
Direct vs indirect composite	– Direct and indirect composite restorations have similar performance and longevity [24]

HR hazard ratio, *AFR* annual failure rate

fail [60], corroborating with a systematic review that observed caries as the main reason for the failure of posterior restoration in primary teeth, independently of restorative material [9]. On the other hand, considering anterior composite restorations in permanent teeth, caries has a low contribution in failures in a systematic review [11], probably due to a low incidence of caries in the anterior region compared to posterior teeth. Practice-based studies have already corroborated these findings [37, 61, 62].

10.1.1.2 Fracture

Tooth/restoration fracture has been highlighted as the main reason for failure in anterior teeth. In a systematic review that evaluated the longevity of anterior restoration, the fracture (tooth/restoration) was the most common reason for failure among all studies [11], with rates varying from 25 to 100% of all failures observed in the included studies.

Bruxism of parafunctional habits probably plays a significant role in the fracture of the tooth or restorations via tooth-restoration complex fatigue, resulting in a fracture as a long-term outcome. In addition to the complex etiopathogenic mechanisms of bruxism, which hinder its correct diagnosis, in general, studies do not use reliable instruments for their assessment. Also, quite often, studies excluded bruxism patients. Restorations performed in participants with severe tooth wear presented negative findings when compared to participants without bruxism habits in a clinical study with patients with severe tooth wear [63]. Indeed, when restorations are placed in individuals presenting bruxism symptoms, more failures due to fracture could occur [64]. In a practice-based study, when patients showed "occlusal-stress," there was a 2.6-fold risk of failure than in individuals with "no risk" [8].

10.1.1.3 Esthetic Demand

Modern society has increased the demand for esthetics [65]. Especially the anterior teeth must be well-aligned and white, which impacts the oral health-related quality of life [66]. The high visibility and the importance of the smile's appearance expose the anterior restorations to a greater risk of undergoing interventions due to esthetic demands. In this region, small marginal pigmentations observed with the natural degradation of the hybrid layer or small natural changes in color or shape resulting from the natural aging of composites can result in early interventions in these restorations. Especially in patients who exhibit a high esthetic demand. Unlike the posterior region, where color changes appear to be less important [49]. It is clear that these changes are linked to factors related to patients and may depend on cultural and contextual factors of these individuals, which are incredibly subjective.

Upper front teeth restorations exhibited a higher risk for failure when compared with lower front teeth, especially in young patients [37]. Color alterations, marginal mismatch, and surface staining are some of the motifs for patients to require replacement of their veneer restorations [67]. However, for posterior teeth, the esthetic demand is a less important factor to some patients. When evaluating restorations after 27 years in clinical service, the ones carried out with chemical-cured resin composite (which presents accelerate deterioration of color match linked to the non-color stable initiators of the peroxide-initiated curing mechanism) were 59% non-acceptable to the researchers who evaluated these restorations, while only 6.3% of light-cured materials were classified as non-acceptable. However, these restorations were not classified as a failure because no patients requested replacement of non-acceptable color restoration, which were in function [49].

10.1.2 Factors Involved in Esthetic Restorations Failure

Whereas most of the attention in the clinical studies in restorative dentistry is given to the restoration's longevity and the failure causes, it is of utmost importance to study all the factors affecting the restoration's failure. I this context, even if most clinicians give quite some importance to the dental material and dental techniques, factors related to the characteristics of the patient, operator, and tooth are critical in assessing the long-term survival of restorations [10]. Also, population studies found that socioeconomic and demographic factors influenced the choice of restorative materials, the patients' risk status, and, consequently, the longevity of the dental restorations [58].

10.1.2.1 Tooth Factors

Restoration survival depends on several clinical-related factors for their longevity, including the tooth position in the dental ark, tooth type, cavity size, previous endodontic treatment, and substrate type [3, 10, 27].

Restorations in premolars have shown better survival results than those placed in molars, and the explanations are related to higher masticatory forces observed in the molar region [8, 10, 38, 68–70]. After 10 years, general practitioners' restorations have a hazard ratio of 2.3 to fail in molar than premolar [36]. Similar results have been reported in other studies [8, 10, 38, 68–70]. After 27 years, class II restorations in molars presented a failure risk almost 5 higher than premolars [49]. However, some studies did not find significant differences [45, 71]. For restoration in anterior teeth, failures were more frequent in upper central incisors and upper canines, when evaluating both children and adults in a practice-based study [37].

The increase in the number of surfaces involved in the restorations has been associated with a higher risk of failure [10, 36, 38, 72]. Posterior restorations fail 3.3 times more often in teeth with fewer than 2 remaining walls than those with 4 [73]. For premolars, each surface included in the restoration introduces a hazard risk of 1.5, while for molars, the risk is 1.24 [27]. Opdam et al. [38] estimate that each restored surface's addition leads to an increased 40% risk of failure. Similarly, it was reported that every extra missing wall increases the failure risk from 30 to 40% [74]. Thus, class II restorations present a higher risk than Class I. Also, class III restorations tend to fail less than other anterior restorations types [11]. Collares et al. [37] observed a high-risk of failure in anterior restorations with three or more involved surfaces (Class IV) than class III restoration, highlighting that restoration size is an important predictor of failure risk also in anterior teeth.

Glass ionomer cement sandwich-type restorations are frequently used to perform indirect pulp protection in deep caries lesions. Using a GIC liner or base under composite resin restorations has shown divergent results in the literature. In several studies, the use of an intermediate GIC liner negatively influenced the restorations' survival, resulting in more fracture of composite resin [10, 27, 38, 75, 76]. An AFR of 3.8% was observed for class II restorations with glass ionomer bases while observing an AFR of 1.4% for restorations without a base material [38]. In opposite, other studies observed no effect on restoration longevity when using GIC liners [44, 68, 77]. The thickness and type of glass ionomer cement used could explain the different results observed [10, 44]. Therefore, there is no consensus in the literature about the influence of GIC under composite restorations.

The endodontic treatment represents a challenging situation for restoration longevity in both anterior and posterior teeth. The significant loss of dental structure in these teeth could be related to the main reason for reducing the success rate. A 13-year clinical trial comparing restorations in vital and endodontic treated teeth observed AFR of 0.08 and 1.78%, respectively [40]. An AFR of 4.9% was observed in vital teeth and 9.8% in non-vital teeth in evaluating anterior composite veneers. Veneers made in non-vital teeth had a higher risk of failure (HR 2.78; 95% CI 1.02–7.56) over time compared to those made in vital teeth [39].

The selective carious tissue removal of soft dentine has also been discussed. It is important to consider that selective caries removal decreases the risk of pulp exposition [41] and can improve the longevity of restorations [42]. A 5-years randomized trial observed that selective caries removal to soft dentin in deep caries did not affect the restoration survival when compared to stepwise excavation [43]. A systematic review observed that selective caries removal have similar results in restoration longevity than stepwise excavation and result in fewer pulp complications [42]. Similar results were observed in a multicenter clinical trial considering primary posterior teeth. The longevity of restorations was similar between non-selective and selective carious tissue removal over 33 months [78]; but a systematic review with a limited number of included articles with a high risk of bias have observed that—in primary teeth—selective caries removal decrease the restoration longevity [79]. Thus, for primary teeth, no definitive conclusion about the influence of selective caries removal on restoration longevity can be performed.

10.1.2.2 Patients' Related Factors

The focus of a vast number of clinical trials investigating the survival of restorations is limited to comparisons between technic or materials [80, 81] while patients-related factors are not investigated. The contribution to patient-related factors on restoration survival cannot be ignored [11, 27, 28]. When patients are not mainly selected for inclusion criteria in clinical trials, some studies have observed that failures are linked to certain participants, independently of restorative material used [82]. Similar results are observed in epidemiological studies where caries is the central factor in explaining the failure and replacement of dental restorations [83, 84]. Corroborating, a birth cohort study, observed that unsatisfactory restorations at 24 years were more prevalent in individuals that presented a high number of decayed teeth at 15 years [58].

Caries risk of patients has been associated with higher restorations failure. Restorations placed in the high-risk group showed a lower survival rate than the low-risk group after 5 and 12 years. Considering 12 years of evaluation, AFR was 4.2% in the high-risk group and 0.9% in the low caries risk group [45]. In a clinical trial, corroborating that after 30 years, 64% of restorations that failed due to secondary caries were observed in the high-risk group [71]. A review observed that caries risk was associated with decreased restoration survival, including amalgam and composite resin [28]. In a cohort study evaluating posterior restorations (composite or amalgam), it was observed that individuals who had a higher trajectory of caries during their life were more likely to present failed restorations in adult life [47]. In another cohort study, in children at the age 12, the chances of presenting unsatisfactory restorations were 5.3 higher in children at high-risk for untreated dental caries in the permanent dentition than children at low risk. If the parents have received orientation from professionals on preventing caries development in their offspring, the children exhibited a 91.0% less chance of having an unsatisfactory restoration than children whose parents never received information [46]. Decayed, missing, filled teeth-surfaces (DMFT-S) have been used to evaluate caries experience, even as the component D of DMFT. Also, the number of the previous restoration was used to access caries risk. However, the use of a cumulative indicator could overestimate the caries risk. Therefore, identifying high-caries risk patients when the restoration is placed may provide a reasonable estimate, such as the lesion activity assessment [85].

Bruxism and parafunctional habits have been reported as factors that overload the restorations and increases the likelihood of restoration/teeth failure due to fatigue. Fracture of restorations is frequently reported as the second main reason for restorations failure. Fracture is the main failure of patients with habits of grinding and clenching teeth [8]. 70% of the restoration's fractures occurred in patients with the parafunctional habit in a long-term follow-up (30 years) [71]. Patients with bruxism were also associated with a 37-fold more failed restoration or catastrophic fracture occurred whether the teeth presented root canal treatment [40]. In a practice-based retrospective study that evaluated the survival of resin composite restorations in posterior teeth, individuals with high occlusal-stress displayed three times higher risk to failure than individuals with low occlusal-stress; moreover, individuals with occlusal-stress and caries risk showed a cumulative effect and eight times more failures than individuals no risk [8].

Instruments for assessing bruxism habits used in studies that evaluate restorative materials are not objective, and they do not present standardized cutoff points, which limit their inference [10]. The most recent International Consensus [86] proposed a system for evaluating bruxism, considering that possible bruxism during sleep is based only on the author's report (report of patients), probable sleep bruxism (with clinical inspection such as the presence of tooth wear), and definitive sleep bruxism (based on instrumental assessment, such as polysomnographic). Furthermore, bruxism's etiology is considered to be multifactorial, and several underlying mechanisms may play a role in triggering and perpetuating events [87].

Post-operative sensitivity was one of the causes of patient-related failures in the first clinical studies evaluating composite restorations; however, such aspect is not observed in modern studies, primarily due to the improvements in adhesive systems [88] and restorative technique [89]. Several studies have found that participant's age significantly influences restoration longevity

[37, 90, 91]. The explanations are directed to the influence of age in other co-variables like dental caries, patient cooperation, among others, and it is not recommended to be considered as an isolated factor [5]. Caries activity has been reported to be the more frequent reason for making a dental restoration in the young population. Consequently, these restorations would be subject to higher risk due to individual factors. A study that followed 4355 restorations placed by 115 dentists in the Public Dental Health Service in Denmark observed that posterior composite resin restorations placed in children presented more likely to fail than those placed in the adolescent group [90].

10.1.2.3 Socioeconomic Status

Limited studies have investigated the influence of socioeconomic variables and their influence on the longevity of composite restorations. Most studies evaluating the longevity of restorations are carried out in private dental clinics or are performed under high control in randomized clinical trials, excluding patients with high-caries risk [10]. Frequently only individuals with high socioeconomic status are included. However, the findings of studies that investigate the influence of socioeconomic status suggest that it influences dental restorations survival via dental caries. One study carried out in a birth cohort investigate the influence of socioeconomic trajectory in the life course and found more unsatisfactory restorations in the low trajectory group. Individuals who always lived in the poorest stratus presented more failures than those who lived in the wealthiest layer [58]. A more recent follow-up of this cohort reported that posterior restorations' failures were significant associated with socioeconomic status at age 30, with a prevalence ratio of 2.21 (95% CI 1.19–4.09) in low-income tertile [47]. In the same way, a recent study assessing restorations performed in the Brazilian public oral health service found that people with lower access to public services presented lower survival rates of composite restorations [92]. A practice-based study also observed that restorations performed by clinicians located in the more deprived region presented higher AFR than those found in areas of medium and high socioeconomic status [48]. Some studies have corroborated with the discussion of the influence of socioeconomic and behavioral factor on the survival of composite resins [93–96].

10.1.2.4 Restorative Material

Although *in vitro* studies have found considerable differences between the properties of commercially available restorative materials [97, 98], these findings are limited in predicting the clinical behavior of restorations [76]. In fact, in vitro and clinical studies have presented contradictory evidence of direct restorations' clinical performance in posterior teeth [24]. Perhaps differences observed in laboratory tests will take decades to be observed clinically [17]. Yet, the differences can be so minor in clinical outcomes that they may not be statistically significant [71]. For posterior teeth, a retrospective study with data from one dentist's private clinical practice followed two types of composites for long periods. No differences in performances were observed 17 years; however, after 22 years of follow-up, midfilled (70 vol% inorganic filler loading) composite showed superior performance than minifilled (55 vol% inorganic filler loading) [17]. Similar tendencies were observed to anterior restorations: only after 10 years of follow-up significative differences between restorative composites were clinically observed [61].

Another study that retrospectively evaluated for up to 20 years the longevity of restorations placed by one operator under rubber dam isolation and patients with regular check-up visits did not find differences between the composites placed in posterior teeth [99]. Similarly, after 30 years of another controlled trial, no differences between composite resins placed with chemical-cured and light-cured resin composite were observed regarding survival rate. Thus, to compare the clinical survival of restorations is necessary long-term studies. Moreover, these studies' results are with materials that were developed decades ago and are expected to be inferior to the composite resins recently developed.

A wide number of composite materials have been introduced in the market, and the clinical trials' design to compare these new materials present few years of follow-up. The main modification in the inorganic formulation of composites was the introduction of nanofiller composites. These materials were created to provide superior polish and gloss retention. A randomized 10-years trial of class II nanohybrid and conventional hybrid resin composite observed an overall AFR of 1.9% and no significant difference between the composites [100]. In another study, the overall success rate was 100% after 6 years of clinical evaluation for nanohybrid and hybrid composite [101]. At 8 years, the success rate was 98.5%, with no differences observed between materials [102].

A recent development in resin composite technology was the introduction of "bulk-fill" resin composites. Bulk-fill composites can be cured in up to 4 or 5 mm layers and include both low as high viscosity materials. A randomized clinical trial compared to class I and II restorations compared flowable bulk-filled resin composite (in increments up to 4 mm as needed to fill the cavity and 2 mm short of the occlusal cave surface with the occlusal part completed with nanohybrid resin composite) and resin composite-only placed in 2 mm increments. After 5 years of evaluation, bulk-filled presented an AFR of 1.1% and the resin composite-only restorations of 1.3%, with no significant differences detected between the materials [102].

Although the comparisons of direct and indirect composite restorations have similar performance and longevity [24], other factors related to the restorative technique have been reported to influence the clinical performance of composite materials. Adhesive systems are frequently evaluated in Class V restorations and also influenced the longevity of these restorations [103], even though, for anterior restorations, the degradation of the hybrid layer could affect more the esthetics, while such aspect seems not to be relevant for posterior composite restorations [88, 104, 105]. Regarding longevity or restorations, the gold standard dental adhesive technique is the use of a mild two-step, self-etch adhesive system with selective phosphoric acid enamel etching [50] and bevel are not indicated because they does not affect the clinical performance [34]. Moreover, the use of rubber dam isolation does not seem to affect the longevity of restorations, as long as it is applied effectively with cotton rolls and suction devices. Although some studies have observed better performances of restorations applied under rubber dam isolation [9, 34], the evidence shows that restorations placed using cotton rolls and suction device can also survive for long periods [49] and the use of appropriate suction device and working with the aid of a dental nurse are even more important for achieving good isolation from humidity in case rubber dam is not used.

10.1.2.5 Operator

Dentist-linked factors, such as operator skills, are considered important factors that influenced the survival of composite resin restorations [5]. Although a wide part of results is explained solely on the training level and accuracy of work, the decision-making process also can influence restoration survival and could combine as a complex process, ranging among clinicians according to co-variables, such as the type of practice, reimbursement system, competition environment among dentists, patients' views and opinions, and cultural aspects.

The dentists are the ones who place the restorations, those who evaluate them, and, ultimately, decide when the restoration needs to be changed. Variability on diagnostic and decision-making has been elevated among dentists that frequently adopt an invasive approach to intervene in restorations, especially when they were performed by other professionals [13]. Invasive behavior toward restoration replacement results in a decrease in the survival of restoration. Chisini et al. [106] observed that the decision-making of dentists was influenced by patient skin color. Clinicians choose more to replace ill-adapted restoration in white patients while they decide not to intervene in restoration from dark-skinned individuals [106]. Dentists frequently choose to replace restorations with a small sign of marginal degradation or staining because they then confound with secondary caries. After 27 years of follow-up on posterior chemical-cured resin composite with the high color changed (classified as non-acceptable research evaluators) were maintained in function and classified as satisfactory to the patients [49]. Even secondary caries kept restricted in the enamel can be maintained and treated with non-operative treatments [107], and the repair can—preferably—choose if operative treatment is required.

Despite clinical studies with trained and calibrated operators maybe not observe significant associations between operator and success, practice-based studies have observed that age, country of qualification, and employment status of the operator could influence the survival of restoration [5]. Data from Washington dental service observed that restorations placed by efficient dentists survive almost 5 months more than restorations performed by inefficient dentists, and no differences between the restorations were observed when efficient dentists performed than [108]. Similarly, the longevity of restorations placed by more experienced clinicians was better than those placed for less experienced ones [109]. Restorations placed by the dentist with less practice workload presented a success rate of about twice than those slightly busy clinicians [110]. A geospatial analysis carried out in Canada observed more aggressive treatment choices were performed by dentists who feel under great competitive pressure and in low dentist density areas [111]. Therefore, all these issues and the differences in the decision-making process on judging restorations intensification the risk for replacement restorations and decrease the survival rates.

10.2 Repairing Esthetic Composite Restorations

Patients that changed the dentist have an increased chance to replace their restorations [93–96]. In fact, a cross-sectional study that included 194 dentists of the Dental Practice-Based Research Network observed that the decision to repair defective restoration instead to replace is influenced by who place the original one: clinicians are less demanding when evaluating their work [13]. The decision to replace a restoration relies on the dentist's clinical expertise rather than on strict criteria. Thus, dentists adopt different approaches (repair or replacement) in cases of imperfect restorations [112], although the literature presents a consensus that, when possible, repaired restorations presents benefits and are more cost-effective than replacement [16].

10.2.1 Long-Term Survival and Reasons for Failures of Repaired Restorations

Replacement of a failed restoration is still one of the most frequent treatments performed in dental practice [113]. While most dentists state to perform repairs, and the vast majority of dental schools teach repairs, the proportion of truly repaired restorations is still very low [16]. A clinical trial assessed the longevity of repaired restorations and showed similar longevity than replaced restorations after 12 years of follow-up [15]. Repaired and replaced restorations presented similar behavior in marginal adaptation, marginal stain, teeth sensitivity, anatomic form, and luster parameter, although roughness was significative was significantly worse in the group of repaired restorations [15].

Casagrande et al. [114] estimated the reduction in AFR when repaired restorations were not considered as a "true failure" and observed that repair increases the longevity of direct posterior restorations. When repair was not considered as a failure, the survival of restoration changed from 83.1 (AFR = 3.6%) to 87.9% (ARF = 2.5%) at 5 years and from 65.9 (AFR = 4.1%) to 74.6% (AFR = 2.9%) at 10 years of follow-up. Reduction of AFR from 1.83 to 0.72% in composite resins repaired restorations after 12 years of follow-up was observed in another study [115]. A study that follows for 22 years posterior composite restorations performed by one dentist observed that a reduction from 1.9 to 0.7% on AFR when restorations repaired were not considered as failures [10, 17].

A study that evaluated 880 restorations placed in posterior and anterior teeth observed that repair increases the survival of restorations even after previous repairs or replacements [116]. A recent long-term practice-based clinical study carried out in a private dental practice followed class III and class IV for 15 years, and veneer restorations for 10 years. For class III and class IV restoration, AFR was 2.9%, and for veneers 9.2% when the repair was considered as failure. When repair was not considered as failure, class III and IV presented an AFR of 2.4% and veneers of 6.3% [117]. Thus, direct comparisons between the treatments (repair and replacement) presented comparable results.

In this way, secondary caries was the main reason for failure in both repaired and replaced restorations [15] while Opdam et al. [115] reported tooth fracture as the main reason for failure in the repaired restorations (41.1%) followed by dental caries (24.2%) [115]. These two reasons are the same observed for non-repaired restorations both in permanent [8, 10] and primary teeth [9].

10.2.2 Factors Involved in Repaired Restorations Failure

Regarding the main reasons for failures, studies have shown, in general, that the same factors known for non-repaired restorations seem to influence repaired restorations as well. Casagrande et al. [114] found that endodontic treatment, molar teeth, use of a prosthesis, and age were important risk factors for restoration failure. On the other hand, in one study, only sex was reported as associated as a risk factor to failure in repaired restorations, in which women presented a risk of failure twice higher when compared to men [115]. Cox regression analysis in a practice-based study found that class III and IV restorations placed in the upper jaw had a higher risk for failure compared to the lower jaw. Central incisors also had a higher failure risk for failed repaired restorations. Also, the type of composite influenced the survival rates [117]. The presence of endodontic treatment is a factor associated with a higher risk of failure for both repaired or replaced restorations [116].

10.2.3 Repairing Benefits Over Replacing Restorations

The comparison of the survival of replaced versus repaired restoration may be unfair. A repaired restoration is comprised mostly of the older and aged part of a restoration. It presents already signs of fatigue, differently from a replaced filling that is entirely new. Thus, a repaired and older restoration may fail before the replaced one. But even in this case, the survival of the original restoration is increased, and the removal of tooth tissue is postponed, which could be the main direct benefits. If the repaired restoration fails, the replacement is indicated and can be carried out without further problems. Repair is considered an approach of minimal intervention dentistry, being an alternative to easy, fast, and low-cost treatment [16]. The clinical time spent to replace a restoration is reported to be higher than the time required to repair the same restoration. Additionally, the repair of restoration seems to be more cost-effective than replacement, and thus repairs are drawn as an important strategy for public health services [16].

10.2.4 When Repairing Is Not a Solution?

Repair of defective restorations is not always possible. Like this, the Academy of Operative Dentistry European Section has indicated the restoration replacement when (a) restoration has unaccepted qualities (deterioration/secondary caries); (b) repair is contraindicated; (c) benefits of replacement are less than possible harm; (d) prospects for an acceptable clinical outcome are favorable; and (e) patient consents [118].

10.3 Replacing Esthetic Composite Restorations

As previously discussed, composites have shown considerable improvements since their introduction in the 1960s. Due to the improvement of the properties of the material, nowadays, most of the failures are related to factors related to the patient and the operator. When small changes in color, shape, or fractures are observed, repair should always be the first choice. However, in some situations where the remaining restoration is integrally degraded, replacement of the restoration can be indicated.

10.3.1 Restorations Do Not Last Forever

Composite resin restorations are materials that, like any other, present aging over time. The degradation of the hybrid layer and its respective pigmentation are the main surface changes in the medium term; together with small changes in surface roughness, they can be overcome with surface finishing and polishing. However, this marginal degradation or marginal staining cannot be mistakenly interpreted as secondary caries. Limited time is used to teach secondary caries diagnosis in dental schools and this fact could be a contributor for the lack of consensus among dentists regarding the interventions on restorative. Considering that criteria for repair/replacement are not clear among dentists, [118] suggest a shift from "in doubt, take it out" toward "as a last resort take it out" after considering monitoring, refurbishment, and repair as the first treatment options.

10.3.2 Aspects That Can Increase the Longevity of Esthetic Composite Restorations

Composite restorations have shown excellent survival rates on anterior and posterior teeth. Due to materials improvements overtime, current materials' properties have revelated a minor influence on the survival of composites in clinical studies. When hybrid or nanohybrid composites are used, low AFR could be expected. To improve the longevity of these restorations, patient-related factors and operators are fundamental. Therefore, restorations should be carried out in a health promotion environment, emphasizing preventive practices. The adoption of healthy behaviors by patients will consequently led to "healthy" restorations, increasing the longevity of treatments. The adoption of minimally invasive dentistry for the management of deteriorated restorations, such as refurbishment or repair restorations, should be considered in routine practice. In this way, dentists should react less in front of small defects of restorations, indicating replacements only when other alternatives are not plausible.

References

1. Demarco FF, Baldissera RA, Madruga FC, Simoes RC, Lund RG, Correa MB, Cenci MS. Anterior composite restorations in clinical practice: findings from a survey with general dental practitioners. J Appl Oral Sci. 2013;21:497–504.
2. Nascimento GG, Correa MB, Opdam N, Demarco FF. Do clinical experience time and postgraduate training influence the choice of materials for posterior restorations? Results of a survey with Brazilian general dentists. Braz Dent J. 2013;24:642–6.
3. Manhart J, Chen H, Hamm G, Hickel R. Buonocore memorial lecture. Review of the clinical survival of direct and indirect restorations in posterior teeth of the permanent dentition. Oper Dent. 2004;29:481–508.
4. Maran BM, de Geus JL, Gutierrez MF, Heintze S, Tardem C, Barceleiro MO, Reis A, Loguercio AD. Nanofilled/nanohybrid and hybrid resin-based composite in patients with direct restorations in posterior teeth: a systematic review and meta-analysis. J Dent. 2020;99:103407.
5. Demarco FF, Collares K, Correa MB, Cenci MS, Moraes RR, Opdam NJ. Should my composite restorations last forever? Why are they failing? Braz Oral Res. 2017;31:e56.
6. Mesko ME, Sarkis-Onofre R, Cenci MS, Opdam NJ, Loomans B, Pereira-Cenci T. Rehabilitation of severely worn teeth: a systematic review. J Dent. 2016;48:9–15.
7. Vetromilla BM, Opdam NJ, Leida FL, Sarkis-Onofre R, Demarco FF, van der Loo MPJ, Cenci MS, Pereira-Cenci T. Treatment options for large posterior restorations: a systematic review and network meta-analysis. J Am Dent Assoc. 2020;151:614–24.
8. van de Sande FH, Opdam NJ, Rodolpho PA, Correa MB, Demarco FF, Cenci MS. Patient risk factors' influence on survival of posterior composites. J Dent Res. 2013;92:78S–83S.
9. Chisini LA, Collares K, Cademartori MG, de Oliveira LJC, Conde MCM, Demarco FF, Correa MB. Restorations in primary teeth: a systematic

review on survival and reasons for failures. Int J Paediatr Dent. 2018;28:123–39.
10. Demarco FF, Correa MB, Cenci MS, Moraes RR, Opdam NJ. Longevity of posterior composite restorations: not only a matter of materials. Dent Mater. 2012;28:87–101.
11. Demarco FF, Collares K, Coelho-de-Souza FH, Correa MB, Cenci MS, Moraes RR, Opdam NJ. Anterior composite restorations: a systematic review on long-term survival and reasons for failure. Dent Mater. 2015;31:1214–24.
12. Elderton RJ. Restorations without conventional cavity preparations. Int Dent J. 1988;38:112–8.
13. Gordan VV, Riley J 3rd, Geraldeli S, Williams OD, Spoto JC 3rd, Gilbert GH, National Dental PCG. The decision to repair or replace a defective restoration is affected by who placed the original restoration: findings from the National Dental PBRN. J Dent. 2014;42:1528–34.
14. Kanzow P, Hoffmann R, Tschammler C, Kruppa J, Rodig T, Wiegand A. Attitudes, practice, and experience of German dentists regarding repair restorations. Clin Oral Investig. 2017;21:1087–93.
15. Estay J, Martin J, Viera V, Valdivieso J, Bersezio C, Vildosola P, Mjor IA, Andrade MF, Moraes RR, Moncada G, Gordan VV, Fernandez E. 12 Years of repair of amalgam and composite resins: a clinical study. Oper Dent. 2018;43:12–21.
16. Kanzow P, Wiegand A, Schwendicke F. Cost-effectiveness of repairing versus replacing composite or amalgam restorations. J Dent. 2016;54:41–7.
17. Da Rosa Rodolpho PA, Donassollo TA, Cenci MS, Loguercio AD, Moraes RR, Bronkhorst EM, Opdam NJ, Demarco FF. 22-Year clinical evaluation of the performance of two posterior composites with different filler characteristics. Dent Mater. 2011;27:955–63.
18. Afrashtehfar KI, Ahmadi M, Emami E, Abi-Nader S, Tamimi F. Failure of single-unit restorations on root filled posterior teeth: a systematic review. Int Endod J. 2017a;50:951–66.
19. Afrashtehfar KI, Emami E, Ahmadi M, Eilayyan O, Abi-Nader S, Tamimi F. Failure rate of single-unit restorations on posterior vital teeth: a systematic review. J Prosthet Dent. 2017b;117:345–53.
20. Ahmed KE, Murbay S. Survival rates of anterior composites in managing tooth wear: systematic review. J Oral Rehabil. 2016;43:145–53.
21. Angeletaki F, Gkogkos A, Papazoglou E, Kloukos D. Direct versus indirect inlay/onlay composite restorations in posterior teeth. A systematic review and meta-analysis. J Dent. 2016;53:12–21.
22. Astvaldsdottir A, Dagerhamn J, van Dijken JW, Naimi-Akbar A, Sandborgh-Englund G, Tranaeus S, Nilsson M. Longevity of posterior resin composite restorations in adults—a systematic review. J Dent. 2015;43:934–54.
23. Beck F, Lettner S, Graf A, Bitriol B, Dumitrescu N, Bauer P, Moritz A, Schedle A. Survival of direct resin restorations in posterior teeth within a 19-year period (1996–2015): a meta-analysis of prospective studies. Dent Mater. 2015;31:958–85.
24. da Veiga AM, Cunha AC, Ferreira DM, da Silva Fidalgo TK, Chianca TK, Reis KR, Maia LC. Longevity of direct and indirect resin composite restorations in permanent posterior teeth: a systematic review and meta-analysis. J Dent. 2016;54:1–12.
25. Heintze SD, Rousson V, Hickel R. Clinical effectiveness of direct anterior restorations—a meta-analysis. Dent Mater. 2015;31:481–95.
26. Moraschini V, Fai CK, Alto RM, Dos Santos GO. Amalgam and resin composite longevity of posterior restorations: a systematic review and meta-analysis. J Dent. 2015;43:1043–50.
27. Opdam NJ, van de Sande FH, Bronkhorst E, Cenci MS, Bottenberg P, Pallesen U, Gaengler P, Lindberg A, Huysmans MC, van Dijken JW. Longevity of posterior composite restorations: a systematic review and meta-analysis. J Dent Res. 2014;93:943–9.
28. van de Sande FH, Collares K, Correa MB, Cenci MS, Demarco FF, Opdam N. Restoration survival: revisiting patients' risk factors through a systematic literature review. Oper Dent. 2016;41:S7–S26.
29. Arbildo-Vega HI, Lapinska B, Panda S, Lamas-Lara C, Khan AS, Lukomska-Szymanska M. Clinical effectiveness of bulk-fill and conventional resin composite restorations: systematic review and meta-analysis. Polymers (Basel). 2020;12:1786.
30. Veloso SRM, Lemos CAA, de Moraes SLD, Do Egito Vasconcelos BC, Pellizzer EP, de Melo Monteiro GQ. Clinical performance of bulk-fill and conventional resin composite restorations in posterior teeth: a systematic review and meta-analysis. Clin Oral Investig. 2019;23:221–33.
31. Azeem RA, Sureshbabu NM. Clinical performance of direct versus indirect composite restorations in posterior teeth: a systematic review. J Conserv Dent. 2018;21:2–9.
32. Rasines Alcaraz MG, Veitz-Keenan A, Sahrmann P, Schmidlin PR, Davis D, Iheozor-Ejiofor Z. Direct composite resin fillings versus amalgam fillings for permanent or adult posterior teeth. Cochrane Database Syst Rev. 2014;3:CD005620.
33. Fron Chabouis H, Smail Faugeron V, Attal JP. Clinical efficacy of composite versus ceramic inlays and onlays: a systematic review. Dent Mater. 2013;29:1209–18.
34. Heintze SD, Rousson V. Clinical effectiveness of direct class II restorations—a meta-analysis. J Adhes Dent. 2012;14:407–31.
35. Laske M, Opdam NJM, Bronkhorst EM, Braspenning JCC, Huysmans M. Risk factors for dental restoration survival: a practice-based study. J Dent Res. 2019;98:414–22.
36. Laske M, Opdam NJM, Bronkhorst EM, Braspenning JCC, Huysmans M. Ten-year survival of class II restorations placed by general practitioners. JDR Clin Trans Res. 2016b;1:292–9.
37. Collares K, Opdam NJM, Laske M, Bronkhorst EM, Demarco FF, Correa MB, Huysmans M. Longevity

of anterior composite restorations in a general dental practice-based network. J Dent Res. 2017;96:1092–9.
38. Opdam NJ, Bronkhorst EM, Roeters JM, Loomans BA. Longevity and reasons for failure of sandwich and total-etch posterior composite resin restorations. J Adhes Dent. 2007;9:469–75.
39. Coelho-de-Souza FH, Goncalves DS, Sales MP, Erhardt MC, Correa MB, Opdam NJ, Demarco FF. Direct anterior composite veneers in vital and non-vital teeth: a retrospective clinical evaluation. J Dent. 2015;43:1330–6.
40. Lempel E, Lovasz BV, Bihari E, Krajczar K, Jeges S, Toth A, Szalma J. Long-term clinical evaluation of direct resin composite restorations in vital vs. endodontically treated posterior teeth—retrospective study up to 13 years. Dent Mater. 2019;35:1308–18.
41. Barros M, De Queiroz Rodrigues MI, Muniz F, Rodrigues LKA. Selective, stepwise, or nonselective removal of carious tissue: which technique offers lower risk for the treatment of dental caries in permanent teeth? A systematic review and meta-analysis. Clin Oral Investig. 2020;24:521–32.
42. Hoefler V, Nagaoka H, Miller CS. Long-term survival and vitality outcomes of permanent teeth following deep caries treatment with step-wise and partial-caries-removal: a systematic review. J Dent. 2016;54:25–32.
43. Jardim JJ, Mestrinho HD, Koppe B, de Paula LM, Alves LS, Yamaguti PM, Almeida JCF, Maltz M. Restorations after selective caries removal: 5-year randomized trial. J Dent. 2020;99:103416.
44. van de Sande FH, Rodolpho PA, Basso GR, Patias R, da Rosa QF, Demarco FF, Opdam NJ, Cenci MS. 18-Year survival of posterior composite resin restorations with and without glass ionomer cement as base. Dent Mater. 2015;31:669–75.
45. Opdam NJ, Bronkhorst EM, Loomans BA, Huysmans MC. A 12-Year survival of composite vs. amalgam restorations. J Dent Res. 2010;89:1063–7.
46. Cumerlato C, Demarco FF, Barros AJD, Peres MA, Peres KG, Morales Cascaes A, de Camargo MBJ, da Silva Dos Santos I, Matijasevich A, Correa MB. Reasons for direct restoration failure from childhood to adolescence: a birth cohort study. J Dent. 2019;89:103183.
47. Collares K, Opdam NJ, Peres KG, Peres MA, Horta BL, Demarco FF, Correa MB. Higher experience of caries and lower income trajectory influence the quality of restorations: a multilevel analysis in a birth cohort. J Dent. 2018;68:79–84.
48. Laske M, Opdam NJ, Bronkhorst EM, Braspenning JC, Huysmans MC. Longevity of direct restorations in Dutch dental practices. Descriptive study out of a practice based research network. J Dent. 2016a;46:12–7.
49. Pallesen U, van Dijken JW. A randomized controlled 27 years follow up of three resin composites in class II restorations. J Dent. 2015b;43:1547–58.
50. Van Meerbeek B, Peumans M, Poitevin A, Mine A, Van Ende A, Neves A, De Munck J. Relationship between bond-strength tests and clinical outcomes. Dent Mater. 2010;26:e100–21.
51. Montagner AF, Sande FHV, Muller C, Cenci MS, Susin AH. Survival, reasons for failure and clinical characteristics of anterior/posterior composites: 8-year findings. Braz Dent J. 2018;29:547–54.
52. Brunthaler A, Konig F, Lucas T, Sperr W, Schedle A. Longevity of direct resin composite restorations in posterior teeth. Clin Oral Investig. 2003;7:63–70.
53. Askar H, Krois J, Gostemeyer G, Bottenberg P, Zero D, Banerjee A, Schwendicke F. Secondary caries: what is it, and how it can be controlled, detected, and managed? Clin Oral Investig. 2020;24:1869–76.
54. Machiulskiene V, Campus G, Carvalho JC, Dige I, Ekstrand KR, Jablonski-Momeni A, Maltz M, Manton DJ, Martignon S, Martinez-Mier EA, Pitts NB, Schulte AG, Splieth CH, Tenuta LMA, Ferreira Zandona A, Nyvad B. Terminology of Dental Caries and Dental Caries Management: consensus report of a workshop organized by ORCA and Cariology Research Group of IADR. Caries Res. 2020;54:7–14.
55. Sheiham A. Dietary effects on dental diseases. Public Health Nutr. 2001;4:569–91.
56. Moynihan PJ, Kelly SA. Effect on caries of restricting sugars intake: systematic review to inform WHO guidelines. J Dent Res. 2014;93:8–18.
57. Peres MA, Sheiham A, Liu P, Demarco FF, Silva AE, Assuncao MC, Menezes AM, Barros FC, Peres KG. Sugar consumption and changes in dental caries from childhood to adolescence. J Dent Res. 2016;95:388–94.
58. Correa MB, Peres MA, Peres KG, Horta BL, Barros AJ, Demarco FF. Do socioeconomic determinants affect the quality of posterior dental restorations? A multilevel approach. J Dent. 2013;41:960–7.
59. Alonso V, Darriba IL, Caserio M. Retrospective evaluation of posterior composite resin sandwich restorations with Herculite XRV: 18-year findings. Quintessence Int. 2017;48:93–101.
60. Trachtenberg F, Maserejian NN, Tavares M, Soncini JA, Hayes C. Extent of tooth decay in the mouth and increased need for replacement of dental restorations: the New England Children's amalgam trial. Pediatr Dent. 2008;30:388–92.
61. Baldissera RA, Correa MB, Schuch HS, Collares K, Nascimento GG, Jardim PS, Moraes RR, Opdam NJ, Demarco FF. Are there universal restorative composites for anterior and posterior teeth? J Dent. 2013;41:1027–35.
62. van Dijken JW, Pallesen U. Fracture frequency and longevity of fractured resin composite, polyacid-modified resin composite, and resin-modified glass ionomer cement class IV restorations: an up to 14 years of follow-up. Clin Oral Investig. 2010;14:217–22.
63. Bartlett D, Sundaram G. An up to 3-year randomized clinical study comparing indirect and direct resin composites used to restore worn posterior teeth. Int J Prosthodont. 2006;19:613–7.

64. Hamburger JT, Opdam NJ, Bronkhorst EM, Kreulen CM, Roeters JJ, Huysmans MC. Clinical performance of direct composite restorations for treatment of severe tooth wear. J Adhes Dent. 2011;13:585–93.
65. Silva FBD, Chisini LA, Demarco FF, Horta BL, Correa MB. Desire for tooth bleaching and treatment performed in Brazilian adults: findings from a birth cohort. Braz Oral Res. 2018;32:e12.
66. Goettems ML, Fernandez MDS, Donassollo TA, Henn Donassollo S, Demarco FF. Impact of tooth bleaching on oral health-related quality of life in adults: a triple-blind randomised clinical trial. J Dent. 2021;105:103564.
67. Alonso V, Caserio M. A clinical study of direct composite full-coverage crowns: long-term results. Oper Dent. 2012;37:432–41.
68. Lindberg A, van Dijken JW, Lindberg M. Nine-year evaluation of a polyacid-modified resin composite/resin composite open sandwich technique in class II cavities. J Dent. 2007;35:124–9.
69. Pallesen U, van Dijken JW, Halken J, Hallonsten AL, Hoigaard R. Longevity of posterior resin composite restorations in permanent teeth in public dental health service: a prospective 8 years follow up. J Dent. 2013;41:297–306.
70. van Dijken JW, Pallesen U. Eight-year randomized clinical evaluation of class II nanohybrid resin composite restorations bonded with a one-step self-etch or a two-step etch-and-rinse adhesive. Clin Oral Investig. 2015;19:1371–9.
71. Pallesen U, van Dijken JW. A randomized controlled 30 years follow up of three conventional resin composites in class II restorations. Dent Mater. 2015a;31:1232–44.
72. Lempel E, Toth A, Fabian T, Krajczar K, Szalma J. Retrospective evaluation of posterior direct composite restorations: 10-year findings. Dent Mater. 2015;31:115–22.
73. Tobi H, Kreulen CM, Vondeling H, van Amerongen WE. Cost-effectiveness of composite resins and amalgam in the replacement of amalgam class II restorations. Community Dent Oral Epidemiol. 1999;27:137–43.
74. Smales RJ, Webster DA. Restoration deterioration related to later failure. Oper Dent. 1993;18:130–7.
75. Andersson-Wenckert IE, van Dijken JW, Kieri C. Durability of extensive class II open-sandwich restorations with a resin-modified glass ionomer cement after 6 years. Am J Dent. 2004;17:43–50.
76. da Rosa Rodolpho PA, Cenci MS, Donassollo TA, Loguercio AD, Demarco FF. A clinical evaluation of posterior composite restorations: 17-year findings. J Dent. 2006;34:427–35.
77. van Dijken JW. Durability of resin composite restorations in high C-factor cavities: a 12-year follow-up. J Dent. 2010;38:469–74.
78. Pereira JT, Knorst JK, Ardenghi TM, Piva F, Imparato JCP, Olegario IC, Hermoza RAM, Armas-Vega ADC, de Araujo FB. Pulp vitality and longevity of adhesive restorations are not affected by selective carious removal: a multicenter clinical trial. Caries Res. 2021;55:55–62.
79. Pedrotti D, Cavalheiro CP, Casagrande L, de Araujo FB, Pettorossi Imparato JC, de Oliveira RR, Lenzi TL. Does selective carious tissue removal of soft dentin increase the restorative failure risk in primary teeth? Systematic review and meta-analysis. J Am Dent Assoc. 2019;150:582–90.
80. Shi L, Wang X, Zhao Q, Zhang Y, Zhang L, Ren Y, Chen Z. Evaluation of packable and conventional hybrid resin composites in class I restorations: three-year results of a randomized, double-blind and controlled clinical trial. Oper Dent. 2010;35:11–9.
81. Yazici AR, Ustunkol I, Ozgunaltay G, Dayangac B. Three-year clinical evaluation of different restorative resins in class I restorations. Oper Dent. 2014;39:248–55.
82. van Dijken JW. Direct resin composite inlays/onlays: an 11 year follow-up. J Dent. 2000;28:299–306.
83. Burke FJ, Cheung SW, Mjor IA, Wilson NH. Restoration longevity and analysis of reasons for the placement and replacement of restorations provided by vocational dental practitioners and their trainers in the United Kingdom. Quintessence Int. 1999;30:234–42.
84. Sunnegardh-Gronberg K, van Dijken JW, Funegard U, Lindberg A, Nilsson M. Selection of dental materials and longevity of replaced restorations in public dental health clinics in northern Sweden. J Dent. 2009;37:673–8.
85. Maltz M, Leal FL, Wagner MB, Zenkner J, Brusius CD, Alves LS. Can we diagnose a patient's caries activity based on lesion activity assessment? Findings from a cohort study. Caries Res. 2020;54:218–25.
86. Lobbezoo F, Ahlberg J, Raphael KG, Wetselaar P, Glaros AG, Kato T, Santiago V, Winocur E, De Laat A, De Leeuw R, Koyano K, Lavigne GJ, Svensson P, Manfredini D. International consensus on the assessment of bruxism: report of a work in progress. J Oral Rehabil. 2018;45:837–44.
87. Lavigne GJ, Khoury S, Abe S, Yamaguchi T, Raphael K. Bruxism physiology and pathology: an overview for clinicians. J Oral Rehabil. 2008;35:476–94.
88. Perdigao J, Dutra-Correa M, Castilhos N, Carmo AR, Anauate-Netto C, Cordeiro HJ, Amore R, Lewgoy HR. One-year clinical performance of self-etch adhesives in posterior restorations. Am J Dent. 2007;20:125–33.
89. Perdigao J, Geraldeli S, Hodges JS. Total-etch versus self-etch adhesive: effect on postoperative sensitivity. J Am Dent Assoc. 2003;134:1621–9.
90. Pallesen U, van Dijken JW, Halken J, Hallonsten AL, Hoigaard R. A prospective 8-year follow-up of posterior resin composite restorations in permanent teeth of children and adolescents in public dental health service: reasons for replacement. Clin Oral Investig. 2014;18:819–27.
91. Soncini JA, Maserejian NN, Trachtenberg F, Tavares M, Hayes C. The longevity of amalgam versus compomer/composite restorations in posterior pri-

mary and permanent teeth: findings from the New England Children's amalgam trial. J Am Dent Assoc. 2007;138:763–72.
92. da Silva Pereira RA, da Silva GR, Barcelos LM, Cavalcanti K, Herval AM, Ardenghi TM, Soares CJ. Practice-based analysis of direct posterior dental restorations performed in a public health service: retrospective long-term survival in Brazil. PLoS One. 2020;15:e0243288.
93. Burke FJ, Lucarotti PS, Holder R. Outcome of direct restorations placed within the general dental services in England and Wales (part 4): influence of time and place. J Dent. 2005a;33:837–47.
94. Burke FJ, Lucarotti PS, Holder RL. Outcome of direct restorations placed within the general dental services in England and Wales (part 2): variation by patients' characteristics. J Dent. 2005b;33:817–26.
95. Lucarotti PS, Holder RL, Burke FJ. Outcome of direct restorations placed within the general dental services in England and Wales (part 3): variation by dentist factors. J Dent. 2005a;33:827–35.
96. Lucarotti PS, Holder RL, Burke FJ. Outcome of direct restorations placed within the general dental services in England and Wales (part 1): variation by type of restoration and re-intervention. J Dent. 2005b;33:805–15.
97. Borba M, Della Bona A, Cecchetti D. Flexural strength and hardness of direct and indirect composites. Braz Oral Res. 2009;23:5–10.
98. Koytchev E, Yamaguchi S, Shin-No Y, Suzaki N, Okamoto M, Imazato S, Datcheva M, Hayashi M. Comprehensive micro-mechanical characterization of experimental direct core build-up resin composites with different amounts of filler contents. Dent Mater J. 2019;38:743–9.
99. Borgia E, Baron R, Borgia JL. Quality and survival of direct light-activated composite resin restorations in posterior teeth: a 5- to 20-year retrospective longitudinal study. J Prosthodont. 2019;28:e195–203.
100. van Dijken JW, Pallesen U. A randomized 10-year prospective follow-up of class II nanohybrid and conventional hybrid resin composite restorations. J Adhes Dent. 2014;16:585–92.
101. Kramer N, Garcia-Godoy F, Reinelt C, Feilzer AJ, Frankenberger R. Nanohybrid vs. fine hybrid composite in extended class II cavities after six years. Dent Mater. 2011;27:455–64.
102. Frankenberger R, Reinelt C, Kramer N. Nanohybrid vs. fine hybrid composite in extended class II cavities: 8-year results. Clin Oral Investig. 2014;18:125–37.
103. Matos TP, Gutierrez MF, Hanzen TA, Malaquias P, de Paula AM, de Souza JJ, Hass V, Fernandez E, Reis A, Loguercio AD. A 18-Month clinical evaluation of a copper-containing universal adhesive in non-carious cervical lesions: a double-blind, randomized controlled trial. J Dent. 2019;90:103219.
104. Opdam NJ, Feilzer AJ, Roeters JJ, Smale I. Class I occlusal composite resin restorations: in vivo post-operative sensitivity, wall adaptation, and microleakage. Am J Dent. 1998a;11:229–34.
105. Opdam NJ, Roeters FJ, Feilzer AJ, Verdonschot EH. Marginal integrity and postoperative sensitivity in class 2 resin composite restorations in vivo. J Dent. 1998b;26:555–62.
106. Chisini LA, Noronha TG, Ramos EC, Dos Santos-Junior RB, Sampaio KH, Faria ESAL, Correa MB. Does the skin color of patients influence the treatment decision-making of dentists? A randomized questionnaire-based study. Clin Oral Investig. 2019;23:1023–30.
107. Schwendicke F, Splieth C, Breschi L, Banerjee A, Fontana M, Paris S, Burrow MF, Crombie F, Page LF, Gaton-Hernandez P, Giacaman R, Gugnani N, Hickel R, Jordan RA, Leal S, Lo E, Tassery H, Thomson WM, Manton DJ. When to intervene in the caries process? An expert Delphi consensus statement. Clin Oral Investig. 2019;23:3691–703.
108. Coppola MN, Ozcan YA, Bogacki R. Evaluation of performance of dental providers on posterior restorations: does experience matter? A data envelopment analysis (DEA) approach. J Med Syst. 2003;27:445–56.
109. Opdam NJ, Loomans BA, Roeters FJ, Bronkhorst EM. Five-year clinical performance of posterior resin composite restorations placed by dental students. J Dent. 2004;32:379–83.
110. McCracken MS, Gordan VV, Litaker MS, Funkhouser E, Fellows JL, Shamp DG, Qvist V, Meral JS, Gilbert GH, National Dental Practice-Based Research Network Collaborative G. A 24-month evaluation of amalgam and resin-based composite restorations: findings from the National Dental Practice-Based Research Network. J Am Dent Assoc. 2013;144:583–93.
111. Ghoneim A, Yu B, Lawrence HP, Glogauer M, Shankardass K, Quinonez C. Does competition affect the clinical decision-making of dentists? A geospatial analysis. Community Dent Oral Epidemiol. 2020;48:152–62.
112. Heaven TJ, Gordan VV, Litaker MS, Fellows JL, Brad Rindal D, Firestone AR, Gilbert GH, National Dental PCG. Agreement among dentists' restorative treatment planning thresholds for primary occlusal caries, primary proximal caries, and existing restorations: findings from the National Dental Practice-Based Research Network. J Dent. 2013;41:718–25.
113. Mjor IA, Shen C, Eliasson ST, Richter S. Placement and replacement of restorations in general dental practice in Iceland. Oper Dent. 2002;27:117–23.
114. Casagrande L, Laske M, Bronkhorst EM, Huysmans M, Opdam NJM. Repair may increase survival of direct posterior restorations—a practice based study. J Dent. 2017;64:30–6.
115. Opdam NJ, Bronkhorst EM, Loomans BA, Huysmans MC. Longevity of repaired restorations: a practice based study. J Dent. 2012;40:829–35.

116. Kanzow P, Wiegand A. Retrospective analysis on the repair vs. replacement of composite restorations. Dent Mater. 2020;36:108–18.
117. van de Sande FH, Moraes RR, Elias RV, Montagner AF, Rodolpho PA, Demarco FF, Cenci MS. Is composite repair suitable for anterior restorations? A long-term practice-based clinical study. Clin Oral Investig. 2019;23:2795–803.
118. Wilson N, Lynch CD, Brunton PA, Hickel R, Meyer-Lueckel H, Gurgan S, Pallesen U, Shearer AC, Tarle Z, Cotti E, Vanherle G, Opdam N. Criteria for the replacement of restorations: Academy of Operative Dentistry European Section. Oper Dent. 2016;41:S48–57.

GPSR Compliance

The European Union's (EU) General Product Safety Regulation (GPSR) is a set of rules that requires consumer products to be safe and our obligations to ensure this.

If you have any concerns about our products, you can contact us on ProductSafety@springernature.com

In case Publisher is established outside the EU, the EU authorized representative is:

Springer Nature Customer Service Center GmbH
Europaplatz 3
69115 Heidelberg, Germany

Batch number: 10731385

Printed by Printforce, the Netherlands